CHALLENGES IN PRIMARY MENTAL HEALTH CARE

This insightful and timely book equips family doctors and other primary healthcare professionals with the knowledge and skills needed to address a diverse range of new and important challenges in the field of primary mental health care, including ongoing impacts from the COVID pandemic, thanatophobia, and end-of-life care, humanitarian and geopolitical catastrophes, and the effects of climate change.

There is an emphasis throughout on the need to encourage and reap the benefits of interdisciplinary collaboration between family doctors and mental health specialists, and across the range of primary care and community workers. Effective primary healthcare relies increasingly on the use of remote consultations, and the book explains how the potential of remote working can be maximized in low-resource settings. The book concludes with a consideration of how to protect and enhance the mental health of primary care workers in the face of these ongoing challenges in care.

Reflecting the expertise of the WONCA Working Party for Mental Health (WWPMH), building on the foundations laid in the 2020 WONCA volume *Global Primary Mental Health Care*, the editors and contributors all have expertise in primary mental health care at the frontline, with backgrounds in family medicine, psychiatry, psychology, and nursing.

WONCA Family Medicine

About the Series

The WONCA Family Medicine series is a collection of books written by world-wide experts and practitioners of family medicine, in collaboration with the *World Organization of Family Doctors* (WONCA). WONCA is a not-for-profit organization and was founded in 1972 by member organizations in 18 countries. It now has 118 Member Organizations in 131 countries and territories with membership of about 500,000 family doctors and more than 90 per cent of the world's population.

How to Do Primary Care Educational Research: A Practical Guide
Mehmet Akman, Valerie Wass, Felicity Goodyear-Smith

ICPC-3 International Classification of Primary Care: User Manual and Classification
Kees van Boven, Huib Ten Napel

Family Medicine in the Undergraduate Curriculum: Preparing Medical Students to Work in Evolving Health Care Systems
Val Wass, Victor Ng

Anxiety and Depression in Primary Care: International Perspectives
Sherina Mohd-Sidik, Felicity Goodyear-Smith

Core Values in Family Medicine: Inspiring Global Change
Anna Stavdal, Johann Agust Sigurdsson, Felicity Goodyear-Smith

Digital Health for Primary Care
Ana Luisa Neves, Lilliana Laranjo

Challenges in Primary Mental Health Care
Christos Lionis, Christopher Dowrick

For more information about this series please visit: https://www.crcpress.com/WONCA-Family-Medicine/book-series/WONCA

CHALLENGES IN PRIMARY MENTAL HEALTH CARE

Models for interdisciplinary collaboration

EDITED BY
Christos Lionis
Christopher Dowrick

CRC Press
Taylor & Francis Group
Boca Raton London New York

CRC Press is an imprint of the
Taylor & Francis Group, an **informa** business

Designed cover image: Shutterstock. Credit: melitas.

First edition published 2026
by CRC Press
2385 NW Executive Center Drive, Suite 320, Boca Raton, FL 33431

and by CRC Press
4 Park Square, Milton Park, Abingdon, Oxon, OX14 4RN

CRC Press is an imprint of Taylor & Francis Group, LLC

ISBN: 978-1-032-75427-7 (hbk)
ISBN: 978-1-032-75426-0 (pbk)
ISBN: 978-1-003-47394-7 (ebk)

DOI: 10.1201/9781003473947

Typeset in Minion Pro
by KnowledgeWorks Global Ltd.

Contents

Foreword by Karen Flegg

Challenges in Primary Mental Health Care is a welcome publication from the World Organization of Family Doctors (WONCA) Working Party on Mental Health. All family doctors will be interested in the approaches in this book, given the large burden of mental health issues in the daily work of family doctors in all countries of the world.

The editors, Christos Lionis (Greece) and Christopher Dowrick (UK), have brought together a diverse range of authors from different countries to contribute their knowledge on this important topic to health professionals in primary healthcare and to their interested patients.

Mental health disorders are on the rise, affecting people of all ages, backgrounds and walks of life, leaving a high burden of mental illness not only on individuals but also on society, with far-reaching implications for healthcare systems, economics, and social cohesion.

As the renowned psychiatrist Viktor Frankl once said, 'When we are no longer able to change a situation, we are challenged to change ourselves.' This book aims to inspire such change, fostering resilience and hope in the face of adversity.

From the silent struggles of mental health to the global challenges posed by the COVID-19 pandemic, climate change, migration, conflicts and wars, it is becoming increasingly evident that mental health crises are not isolated phenomena.

It is forward thinking to include mention of climate change as an urgent existential threat looming over our planet, posing significant challenges to human health, life, and well-being. Anxiety, depression, post-traumatic stress disorder (PTSD), and other mental health conditions are prevalent among those affected by climate-related events.

The world is also witnessing an unprecedented scale of human migration as millions of people leave their homes in search of safety and better opportunities. Forced displacement and the hardships endured during the migration process can inflict severe psychological distress.

The authors state that recognizing the interconnected nature of these challenges is crucial for understanding their impact on mental health and developing comprehensive, holistic approaches to address them.

This book highlights the challenges that call for a more resilient healthcare system that will foster actions toward a major transformation of services for mental health. This in turn will no doubt improve health outcomes and better achieve 'Health for All'.

Karen Flegg, MBBS(Hons), MIntPH, FRACGP, FACRRM, GradDipClinEpi
WONCA President
Associate Professor
Rural Clinical School
College of Science & Medicine
The Australian National University
Canberra, Australia

The Editors

Christos Lionis, MD, PhD, FRCGP(Hon), FESC, FWONCA, is a researcher and academician with a strong interest in primary care and public health. He currently holds the title of Professor Emeritus at the University of Crete. He has been a principal investigator and collaborator on numerous projects funded by the EU and international agencies, and he has published 473 articles that have appeared in PubMed. He also plays an editorial and advisory role with several international journals. Additionally, he is a member of the executive board of various professional organizations, including the WONCA Working Party on Mental Health, where he serves as Chair.

Christopher Dowrick is Emeritus Professor at the University of Liverpool, General Practitioner in Aintree Park Group Practice, and Professorial Research Fellow in the University of Melbourne. He is Past Chair of the WONCA Working Party for Mental Health and provides expert advice to the World Health Organization (WHO) including its mhGAP programme. His research portfolio covers common mental health problems in primary care, with a focus on depression and medically unexplained symptoms. He critiques contemporary emphases on unitary diagnostic categories and medically oriented interventions and highlights the need for socially oriented perspectives. He has developed mental health care for marginalized communities, including asylum seekers and refugees. He is currently exploring the ways in which the creative arts can reduce emotional distress. With WONCA he enables educational interventions for family doctors in Africa, Asia, and Latin America and expands the advocacy skills of family doctors in primary mental health care. He has skills in a wide range of research methodologies, including epidemiology, trial design, qualitative approaches, and theory and strategies for implementation. He has published seven books and over 250 research papers.

Contributors

Abdullah Dukhail AlKhathami
Director Primary Mental
  Health Care Program–MOH
  (Former)
*WONCA Working Party on Mental
  Health (Vice-Chair)*

Marilena Anastasakis
Researcher in Global Public Health
  and Epidemiology
Department of Social Medicine and
  Laboratory Health and Society
School of Medicine
University of Crete
Crete, Greece
*WONCA Working Party on
  Mental Health (Executive
  Member)*

Adekunle Joseph Ariba
Chief Consultant Family
  Physician
Olabisi Onabanjo University
  Teaching Hospital
Sagamu, Nigeria
and
Past Faculty Secretary
Faculty of Family Medicine
National Postgraduate Medical
  College of Nigeria
Ijanikin, Nigeria
*Vice-Chair (Africa Region),
  WONCA Working Party on
  Mental Health (Executive
  Member)*

Laura Canessa
Child and Adolescent Psychiatrist
Associate Professor
Academic Unit of Pediatric Psychiatry
School of Medicine
University of the Republic
Montevideo, Uruguay

Darien Alfa Cipta
Head, Department of Psychiatry
Universitas Pelita Harapan Medical
  School
Tangerang, Indonesia
and
PhD Researcher in DBT and
  Syndemic Prevention
Monash Indonesia School of Public
  Health and Preventive Medicine
Melbourne, Australia
*WONCA Working Party on Mental
  Health (Executive Member)*

Christopher Dowrick
Emeritus Professor of Primary
  Medical Care
University of Liverpool
Liverpool, UK
and
Professorial Research Fellow
University of Melbourne
Melbourne, Australia
*Past Chair of WONCA Working
  Party for Mental Health*

Dyta Ghezhanny William
Department of Psychiatry
Universitas Pelita Harapan
    Medical School
Tangerang, Indonesia
and
PhD Researcher in DBT and
    Syndemic Prevention
Monash Indonesia School of
    Public Health and Preventive
    Medicine
Melbourne, Australia
*WONCA Working Party on Mental
    Health (Executive Member)*

James Jackson
Instructor of Medicine
Harvard Medicine School
Assistant in Medicine
Department of Medicine
Division of Palliative Care and
    Geriatrics
Massachusetts General Hospital
Boston, Massachusetts
*WONCA Working Party on Mental
    Health (Executive Member)*

Christos Lionis
Professor Emeritus of General
    Practice and Primary Health
    Care
Department of Social Medicine and
    Laboratory of Health and Society
School of Medicine
University of Crete
Crete, Greece
*WONCA Working Party on Mental
    Health (Chair)*

Juan Mendive
La Mina Primary Health Care
    Centre–IDIAP Jordi Gol
Barcelona, Spain
European Society for Primary Care
    Gastroenterology (Chair)
and
Associate Professor
University of Barcelona, Spain
*WONCA Working Party on
    Mental Health (Executive
    Member)*

Alfredo de Oliveira Neto
Professor of Primary Health Care
    and Family Medicine
Federal University of Rio de
    Janeiro
Rio de Janeiro, Brazil
*WONCA Working Party on Mental
    Health (Executive Member)*

Ferdinando Petrazzuoli
Center for Primary Health Care
    Research
Department of Clinical
    Sciences
Lund University
Malmö, Sweden
European Rural and Isolated
    Practitioners Association
    (EURIPA) (President)
*WONCA Working Party on Mental
    Health (Executive Member)*

Natasya Reina
Department of Psychiatry
Universitas Pelita Harapan
 Medical School
Tangerang, Indonesia
and
PhD Researcher in DBT and
 Syndemic Prevention
Monash Indonesia School of Public
 Health and Preventive Medicine
Melbourne, Australia
*WONCA Working Party on Mental
 Health (Executive Member)*

Heather L. Rogers
Ikerbasque Associate Professor
Biobizkaia Health Research Institute
Barakaldo, Bizkaia, Spain
and
Ikerbasque Basque Foundation for
 Science
Bilbao, Bizkaia Spain
and
Adjunct Professor
Department of Medicine and
 Surgery
University of the Basque County
Leioa, Bizkaia, Spain
*WONCA Working Party on Mental
 Health (Executive Member)*

Deepika Shaligram
Medical Co-Director of
 Massachusetts Child Psychiatry
 Access Program
Boston Children's Hospital
Harvard Medical School
Boston, Massachusetts

Flávio Dias Silva
Assistant Professor
Family and Community Medicine
 and Psychiatry
Medicine Course
Federal University of Tocantins
Palmas, Brazil
*WONCA Working Party on Mental
 Health (Executive Member)*

Ana B. Pérez Villalva
Family Medicine Physician
ISSSTE
Mexico City, Mexico
*Family Medical Therapist and
 Young Medical Liaison of the
 WONCA Working Party on
 Mental Health (Executive
 Member)*

Introduction
Family medicine facing multiple crises

Christos Lionis and Christopher Dowrick

In today's interconnected world, our collective well-being is profoundly shaped by a complex web of crises. From the silent struggles of mental health to the global challenges posed by health crises introduced by the COVID-19 pandemic, climate change, migration, conflicts, and wars, it is becoming increasingly evident that these crises are not isolated phenomena; instead, they are deeply intertwined, influencing, and exacerbating one another in ways that ripple across societies, economies, and individual lives.

As we grapple with the implications of these crises on people's health and healthcare services, it is crucial to recognize the intricate connections between them and the profound impact they have on mental health and well-being. Similarly, as with physical conditions, mental health cannot be solely viewed within the framework of individual experiences, but is considered as a complex issue linked to broader social and environmental factors [1]. This leads to a deeper understanding of the challenges faced by individuals and communities worldwide, which should be discussed within the healthcare system.

Globally, mental health disorders are on the rise, affecting people of all ages, backgrounds, and walks of life, leaving a high burden of mental illness not only on individuals but also on society, with far-reaching implications for healthcare systems, economics, and social cohesion [2]. A joint report by the European Commission (EC) and Organisation for Economic Co-operation

DOI: 10.1201/9781003473947-1

and Development (OECD) revealed the high burden of mental health illness in adolescents and young adults [3].

Climate change is an urgent existential threat looming over our planet. The disaster of September 2023 following 'Storm Daniel' in Greece and Libya serves as evidence of its impact on communities, populations, and individuals. Rising temperatures, extreme weather events, including deadly floods, and environmental degradation pose significant challenges to human health, life, and well-being. The consequences of climate change, such as loss of livelihoods, displacement, and increased vulnerability, create profound psychological stressors that affect not only mental health but also physical illnesses, including cardiovascular diseases, representing another significant set of public health threats [4]. Anxiety, depression, post-traumatic stress disorder (PTSD), and other mental health conditions are prevalent among those affected by climate-related events [5].

In parallel with the climate crisis, the world is witnessing an unprecedented scale of human migration. Conflicts, political instability, economic disparities, and environmental degradation are driving millions of people to leave their homes in search of safety and better opportunities. Forced displacement and the hardships endured during the migration process can inflict severe psychological distress. Migrants often face isolation, discrimination, and limited access to physical and mental health services, compounding their already challenging circumstances [6]. Numerous examples and experiences can be gained from the war in Ukraine and the ongoing conflicts in the Middle East, Libya, and certain African countries; these are just a few examples of the current violence across the world.

All these combined crises have occurred in a period where the global health crisis has disrupted societies, overwhelmed healthcare systems, and upended lives profoundly. The pandemic's impact on mental health was significant, with increased rates of anxiety, depression, PTSD, loneliness, and grief reported worldwide [7–9]. Isolation, fear, uncertainty, and the socioeconomic consequences of the pandemic have created a perfect storm of psychological challenges leading to a continuum of physical conditions throughout life. Their appearance also highlights the deficiencies of the current healthcare systems, leaving ample room for improvement while seeking better preparedness and resilience.

In this book, we attempt to explore the connections between these combined crises and their serious consequences on mental health, with attempts to unravel the complex tapestry that shapes people's well-being. Recognizing the interconnected nature of these challenges is crucial for understanding their impact on mental health and developing comprehensive, holistic approaches to address them.

Primary care practitioners should adapt their approaches based on individual patient needs, preferences, and values. By incorporating these approaches and acquiring new skills, primary care practitioners can play a vital role in supporting individuals and families affected by the crises and promoting mental health and well-being within their communities.

Is it an easy task? Certainly not; however, this book highlights the challenges that call for a more resilient healthcare system that will foster actions toward a major transformation of its services. The following approaches will be discussed in various chapters of this book.

RECOMMENDATIONS

1. *Integrated Care Approach*: Primary care practitioners can continue to adopt an integrated care approach that considers the interconnected nature of mental health, physical health, and social factors. By incorporating mental health screening and assessment into routine primary care visits, practitioners can identify and address mental health concerns early on. This is a clear message from the latest report issued by the EC and OECD [3]. In some settings, new policies may be needed to emphasize and reward integrated care [10].

2. *Psychoeducation and Behavioural Health*: Primary care practitioners can provide psychoeducation to patients, helping them understand the links between the crises (mental health, climate change, migration, and the pandemic) and their potential impact on their well-being. Promoting behavioural health in primary care refers to mental health and substance use disorders, life stressors, and crises [11]. Primary care physicians need to be equipped and well-trained to provide psychoeducation, and the WONCA Working Party on Mental Health has the skill and capacity to support them in this direction.

3. *Collaborative Care*: The Collaborative Care model is a systematic strategy for treating behavioural health conditions by integrating care managers and psychiatric consultants [12]. This collaborative approach allows for a more holistic assessment, treatment planning, and ongoing support for patients with mental health concerns related to the crises. Achieving this is not an easy target in all settings, and it requires a supportive healthcare policy and sufficient resources.

4. *Community and Cultural Engagement*: Primary care practitioners can actively engage with community organizations, support groups, and local resources related to mental health, climate change, migration, and the pandemic. By connecting patients to relevant community resources, practitioners can help individuals access additional support networks and services. Many paradigms and lessons learned from implementing

collaborative programs can be drawn from both RESTORE [13–15] and EUR-HUMAN [16, 17]. Social prescribing is another effective experience gained from the UK [18]. Recognizing the diverse backgrounds and experiences of patients affected by the crises, primary care practitioners should provide culturally sensitive care. This involves understanding and respecting cultural beliefs, practices, and values that may influence mental health experiences. Creating a safe and inclusive environment that can facilitate open dialogue; trust is a challenging route that requires well-trained primary care practitioners.

5. *Investing in Resilience Building and Self-Compassion for Patients and Practitioners*: Primary care practitioners could promote resilience-building strategies that help patients cope with the challenges posed by the crises. This may include providing resources on stress management, motivational techniques, mindfulness practices, healthy lifestyle choices, and social support systems, with a particular focus on self-compassion. Although we need more studies, there is supportive evidence that reports positive effects of self-compassion intervention in reducing depressive symptoms, anxiety, and stress [19]. Practicing self-care, seeking support, and engaging in professional development activities can assist practitioners in managing their own stress while effectively supporting their patients. This is also a critical concern for stakeholders and governing bodies. It represents an important task for healthcare stakeholders, with recommendations outlined in an EC opinion document [3].

6. *Advocacy and Policy Support*: Primary care practitioners can advocate for policy changes and increased resources for mental health services and support systems. They can offer leadership in communicating the relationship between planetary health and the health of their communities, a compelling message to drive change for sustainability [20]. They can collaborate with local health authorities, policymakers, community organizations, and public health authorities to address systemic barriers, enhance access to mental health care, and implement preventive measures related to the crises. In this context, a focus on training modules to develop leadership skills in young physicians is essential, and examples can be drawn from the WONCA Advocacy project [21].

REFERENCES

1. Compton MT, Shim RS. The social determinants of mental health. Focus. 2015;13(4): 419–425. doi: 10.1176/appi.focus.20150017.
2. Williams N. Are mental health issues increasing? https://www.news-medical.net/ health/Are-Mental-Health-Issues-Increasing.aspx, 2021 Dec 1 (Accessed 19 January 2025).

3. Expert Panel on Effective Ways of Investing in Health (EXPH). Supporting mental health of health workforce and other essential workers. Luxembourg: Publications Office of the European Union, 2021.

4. Romanello M, McGushin A, Di Napoli C, Drummond P, Hughes N, Jamart L, et al. The Lancet countdown on health and climate change: code red for a healthy future. Lancet. 2021 Oct 30;398(10311):1619–1662.

5. Massaza A. https://wellcome.org/news/explained-how-climate-change-affects-mental-health. Wellcome Trust, 2023 (Accessed 13 July 2023).

6. Priebe S, Giacco D, El-Nagib R. Public health aspects of mental health among migrants and refugees: a review of the evidence on mental health care for refugees, asylum seekers and irregular migrants in the WHO European Region. Copenhagen: WHO Regional Office for Europe; 2016. Report No.: 9789289051651.

7. Fan FC, Zhang SY, Cheng Y. Incidence of psychological illness after coronavirus outbreak: a meta-analysis study. J Epidemiol Community Health. 2021 Sep;75(9):836–842.

8. Santabárbara J, Lasheras I, Lipnicki DM, Bueno-Notivol J, Pérez-Moreno M, López-Antón R, et al. Prevalence of anxiety in the COVID-19 pandemic: an updated meta-analysis of community-based studies. Prog Neuropsychopharmacol Biol Psychiatry. 2021 Jul 13;109:110207.

9. Tyler CM, McKee GB, Alzueta E, Perrin PB, Kingsley K, Baker FC, et al. A study of older adults' mental health across 33 countries during the COVID-19 pandemic. Int J Environ Res Public Health. 2021 May 11;18(10):5090.

10. Tsiachristas A, van Ginneken E, Rijken M. Tackling the challenge of multi-morbidity: actions for health policy and research. Health Policy. 2018 Jan;122(1):1–3.

11. Koch U, Bitton A, Landon BE, Phillips RS. Transforming primary care practice and education: lessons from 6 academic learning collaboratives. J Ambulat Care Management. 2017;40(2):125–138.

12. Wang Y, Hu M, Zhu D, Ding R, He P. Effectiveness of collaborative care for depression and HbA1c in patients with depression and diabetes: a systematic review and meta-analysis. Int J Integr Care. 2022 Aug 30;22(3):12.

13. MacFarlane A, O'Donnell C, Mair F, O'Reilly-de Brún M, de Brún T, Spiegel W, et al. Research into implementation strategies to support patients of different origins and language background in a variety of European primary care settings (RESTORE): study protocol. Implement Sci. 2012 Nov 20;7:111.

14. Lionis C, Papadakaki M, Saridaki A, Dowrick C, O'Donnell CA, Mair FS, et al. Engaging migrants and other stakeholders to improve communication in cross-cultural consultation in primary care: a theoretically informed participatory study. BMJ Open. 2016 Jul 22;6(7):e010822.

15. van den Muijsenbergh METC, LeMaster JW, Shahiri P, Brouwer M, Hussain M, Dowrick C, et al. Participatory implementation research in the field of migrant health: sustainable changes and ripple effects over time. Health Expect. 2020 Apr;23(2):306–317.

16. van Loenen T, van den Muijsenbergh M, Hofmeester M, Dowrick C, van Ginneken N, et al. Primary care for refugees and newly arrived migrants in Europe: a qualitative study on health needs, barriers and wishes. Eur J Public Health. 2018 Feb 1;28(1):82–87.

17. Lionis C, Petelos E, Mechili EA, Sifaki-Pistolla D, Chatzea VE, Angelaki A, et al. Assessing refugee healthcare needs in Europe and implementing educational interventions in primary care: a focus on methods. BMC Int Health Hum Rights. 2018 Feb 8;18(1):11.

18. Makanjuola A, Lynch M, Hartfiel N, Cuthbert A, Edwards RT. Prevention of poor physical and mental health through the green social prescribing opening doors to the outdoors programme: a social return on investment analysis. Int J Environ Res Public Health. 2023 Jun 12;20(12):6111.

19. Han A, Tae Hui Kim TH. Effects of self-compassion interventions on reducing depressive symptoms, anxiety, and stress: a meta-analysis. Mindfulness. 2023 June. doi: 10.1007/s12671-023-02148-x.
20. Shergill R, Shrikhande S. Communicating on climate change and health: toolkit for health professionals. Geneva: World Health Organization; 2024
21. Amor SH, Daniels-Williamson T, Fraser-Barclay K, Dowrick C, Gilchrist EC, Gold S, et al. Advocacy training for young family doctors in primary mental health care: a report and global call to action. BJGP Open. 2022 Mar 22;6(1):BJGPO.2021.0163.

SECTION 1

CHAPTER 1

New and emerging mental health challenges

Issues arising from novel threats, including the war in Ukraine and the resulting refugee crisis, as well as climate change

Christos Lionis and Christopher Dowrick

INTRODUCTION

Mamadou is 23 years old. He arrived in your country six months ago. He is seeking asylum, having travelled for many months, and at great financial and personal cost, from the country of his birth. He left his home because severe droughts and desertification meant it was almost impossible to make a living as a pastoral farmer, as his family had done for many generations. He was also at high risk of being arrested and tortured by the new military rulers in his region, as he had been active in protest against them. Now he lives in rundown temporary accommodation near your clinic. He has few friends and very little money. He works washing cars. He believes he contracted COVID at least twice during his migration journey; there was no means of testing nor any way to protect himself from infection from others.

Mamadou consults with you in your clinic because he cannot sleep and keeps crying all the time. He is short of breath on minimal exertion and has pains in his arms and legs. He hears the voices of his parents and sisters, and cannot concentrate on anything.

DOI: 10.1201/9781003473947-3

This chapter begins with a concise introduction to the novel and emerging mental health threats which pose substantial challenges for family physicians and primary care practitioners. Noteworthy among these challenges are climate change, the ongoing COVID-19 pandemic, and the complex migration crisis. Within this chapter, we diligently explore potential frameworks and underlying mechanisms that shed light on how these multifaceted mental health stressors can contribute to the development of mental health disorders.

An integral aspect of this chapter involves a comprehensive analysis of the amalgamated impact stemming from these concurrent compounds of mental health that lead to a combined crisis. Furthermore, the chapter seamlessly transitions into the presentation of illustrative case studies, each serving to provoke insightful ideas, and pragmatic suggestions that can raise effective solutions.

The culmination of this chapter encompasses a compilation of practical recommendations meticulously curated for frontline practitioners. By equipping these healthcare professionals with actionable insights, we aspire to empower them in meeting the formidable mental health challenges posed by the confluence of these intricate factors. Through a judicious amalgamation of theoretical exploration, real-life scenarios, and actionable guidance, this chapter aims to provide a holistic and resourceful framework for navigating the evolving landscape of mental health care.

PARADIGMS OF THE NEW AND EMERGING THREATS

The United Nations (UN) regularly updates its list of countries where peace and security are most at risk. At the time of writing [1], these include:

- The catastrophic humanitarian situation in Gaza, following the recurrence of armed conflict between Israel and Palestine
- The ongoing war in Ukraine, with its consequent ecological and socioeconomic damage
- Civil war and sexual violence in Sudan
- Attacks on civilians in Burkina Faso
- Continued violence in Haiti, displacing one child every minute
- 25 million people caught in a humanitarian crisis in Democratic Republic of the Congo
- The continuing Rohingya refugee crisis on the borders of Myanmar
- Afghanistan, where 'poverty, inequality, and exclusion fuel terrorism'
- And the protracted political, humanitarian, and developmental crisis in Yemen

Climate change is closely linked with many of these threats to peace and security. About 3.5 billion people are living in 'climate hot spots' [2]. Of the 16 countries that are the most climate vulnerable, nine host a UN peace operation: Afghanistan, Central African Republic, Democratic Republic of the Congo, Haiti, Mali, Somalia, Sudan, South Sudan, and Yemen. This demonstrates that the majority of UN peace operations are deployed in contexts that are highly climate exposed.

With further warming, climate change risks will become increasingly complex and more difficult to manage. Multiple climatic and non-climatic risk drivers (including infections and geopolitical conflicts) will interact, resulting in compounding overall risk and risks cascading across sectors and regions [3]. Climate-driven food insecurity and supply instability, for example, are projected to increase with increasing global warming, interacting with non-climatic risk drivers such as competition for land between urban expansion and food production, pandemics, and conflict. Human vulnerability will concentrate in informal settlements and rapidly growing smaller settlements. In rural areas vulnerability will be heightened by high reliance on climate-sensitive livelihoods. Roughly half of the world's population currently experience severe water scarcity for at least part of the year due to a combination of climatic and non-climatic drivers.

In addition to the intense migratory pressures caused by geopolitical conflicts, climate, and weather extremes are increasingly driving displacement in Africa, Asia, North America, and Central and South America, with small island states in the Caribbean and South Pacific being disproportionately affected relative to their small population size.

Climate change and mental health

People living through *extreme weather events* such as floods and storms can be exposed to potentially traumatic events such as witnessing serious injury or death [4]. These problems will often lead to increased psychological distress, including serious mental health problems such as post-traumatic stress disorder (PTSD), depression, or substance use disorders. Extreme weather events can also leading to unemployment, homelessness, or food and water insecurity, which also detrimentally affect mental health.

Climate change is causing *rising temperatures* which can have detrimental impacts on mental health, including hospitalisations for psychiatric disorders, emergency psychiatric visits, and higher rates of suicide [5]. This may be because higher temperatures can worsen mood, leading people to feel more irritable and stressed, and worsen symptoms of mental health problems. Heat can also disrupt sleep, and poor sleep can worsen mental health problems, especially in lower income countries [6].

Poor air quality can negatively impact mental health, in particular depression and anxiety. It is linked with higher risk of acute psychiatric hospital admission and increased mental health service use among people living with psychotic or mood disorders [7].

As well as direct exposure to climate hazards, a growing number of people report psychological reactions related to the prospect of climate change. There are several attempts to describe these reactions, including:

- *Solastalgia*: The inability of finding solace in a familiar landscape due to environmental degradation
- *Ecological grief*: The sense of loss emerging from experiencing environmental degradation
- *Climate anxiety*: A feeling of anxiety in the face of climate change.

One large study of 10,000 children and young people in ten countries found that 45% of respondents said their feelings about climate change negatively impacted their daily functioning [8]. Another study found that negative, climate-related emotions were associated with more symptoms of insomnia and poor mental health [9].

Climate change also increases the risk of *new infectious diseases*, and hence further impacts mental health [10]. Physical and mental health are intrinsically intertwined. Being exposed to higher rates of infectious diseases can have significant detrimental impacts on mental health due to being hospitalized or living with the long-term consequences of severe infection. People living with certain conditions, such as neglected tropical diseases [11], can also face stigma and discrimination.

While most research on climate change and mental health has been conducted in Europe, North America, and Australia, many of the places that are most vulnerable to climate change are in *low- and middle-income* settings. These communities are often most at risk to climate change exposures such as droughts and with fewer resources to adapt to them [12]. Natural disasters in the framework of climate change, including fires and floods, enhance the negative impact on the mental health of people living in these communities [13]. Indigenous communities can be particularly connected and dependent on the natural environment surrounding them, putting them at a higher risk of experiencing poor mental health due to climate change.

For example, members of an Inuit community in Labrador, northern Canada reported that access to land and land-based activities were disrupted due to changes in sea ice, snow, and seasonal temperature, as well as wildlife migration patterns due to warming temperatures. This led to increased family stress, enhanced the possibility of increased drug and alcohol usage, amplified previous traumas and mental health stressors, and increased potential for suicide ideation. As one young man, a local hunter, expressed it:

> *If you take away an internal capability and what makes you feel productive, then those tragedies or that past is still there, and then they're magnified because they come more to the surface because you're not feeling that personal strength.* [14]

However, these communities also possess important forms of local knowledge and expertise that can contribute to their resilience and inform climate change responses in other areas of the world.

COVID-19 pandemic and mental health

One of the biggest global crises in generations, the COVID-19 pandemic, has had severe and far-reaching repercussions for health systems, economies, and societies. Countless people have died or lost their livelihoods. Families and communities have been strained and separated. Children and young people have missed out on learning and socialising. Businesses have gone bankrupt. Millions of people have fallen below the poverty line.

As people grapple with these health, social, and economic impacts, mental health is widely affected [15–17]. Many of us became more anxious, but, for some, COVID-19 has sparked or amplified much more serious mental health problems. People have reported psychological distress and symptoms of depression, anxiety, or post-traumatic stress. And there have been worrying signs of more widespread suicidal thoughts and behaviours [17] including among healthcare workers [18].

A large multi-wave survey across the European Union, investigating the impact of COVID-19 on health and well-being, work, and financial situations, observed a decline in mental well-being since summer 2020, measured using the WHO-5 Well-Being Index, especially among those who had lost their jobs [19]. By spring 2021, the survey showed an overall increase in negative feelings, such as tension/anxiety, loneliness, and feeling downhearted and depressed, across most social groups.

Some groups of people have been affected more than others. Faced with extended school and university closures, young people have been left vulnerable to social isolation and disconnectedness which can fuel feelings of anxiety, uncertainty, and loneliness and lead to affective and behavioural problems. For some children and adolescents, being made to stay at home may have increased the risk of family stress or abuse, which are risk factors for mental health problems. Women have similarly faced greater stress in homes, with an increase in domestic violence during the first year of the pandemic.

The COVID-19 pandemic has had a significant impact on the mental health of individuals worldwide. Frontline physicians, particularly general practitioners and family physicians may experience a surge in the demand for mental health services as more people seek help for anxiety, depression, stress-related disorders, and other mental health conditions. Meeting this increased demand while ensuring timely access to appropriate care can be a challenge [20].

While mental health needs have risen, mental health services have been severely disrupted. This was especially true early in the pandemic when staff and infrastructure were often redeployed to COVID-19 relief. Social measures also prevented people from accessing care at that time. And in many cases, poor knowledge and misinformation about the virus fuelled fears and worries that stopped people from seeking help.

The psychological effects of the pandemic may persist even after the immediate crisis has subsided. Frontline physicians may come across patients experiencing prolonged mental health issues related to grief and loss, trauma, social isolation, financial stress, and the overall disruption caused by the pandemic, often compounded by systemic racism. In Brazil, a young black woman explained why her brother had died after being refused COVID testing:

> *People from the Black population already have very precarious access to health compared to others. In the pandemic, this only worsens because generally, because of structural racism, people will understand that those lives are worthless.* [21]

Addressing and managing these long-term effects will require ongoing support, treatment options, and collaboration with mental health specialists.

Migration crisis and mental health

The Red Cross estimates that more than 100 million people throughout the world have been forced to flee their homes as the impact of climate change, natural disasters, and the number of protracted conflicts has increased. This has more than doubled compared to ten years ago and more than one-third of this group are children. Most displaced people (74%) are hosted in low- and middle-income countries [22].

Asylum seekers and refugees have higher prevalence of psychological morbidity, including depression, anxiety, and PTSD, and functional impairment compared to other migrant groups and local majority populations [23, 24]. These are related to their reasons for leaving their country of origin, their experiences in transit, and their receptions on arrival [22]. Mental health problems are particularly prevalent amongst war refugees with rates of PTSD up to 10 times higher than in the general population [25].

Persistence of mental health problems after resettlement is related to poor socioeconomic conditions, acculturation-related stressors, economic uncertainty, and ethnic discrimination [22, 26]. As a result, they encounter extensive barriers to accessing health care [22] and have substantial unmet mental health needs [8]. Their contact with statutory agencies is often crisis-driven and mediated through voluntary third sector organizations, whose staff – although highly motivated – may lack knowledge and skills in the management of psychosocial distress.

COMPOUND, THEORETICAL FRAMEWORKS, AND CASCADING STRESSORS

To make sense of the interactions between these diverse threats, we usefully turn to the notion of a *syndemic,* proposed by the American anthropologist Merrill Singer. A syndemic is not merely a comorbidity. Syndemics are characterised by biological and social interactions between conditions and states, interactions that increase a person's susceptibility to harm or worsen their health outcomes. Singer argues that a syndemic approach reveals biological and social interactions that are important for prognosis, treatment, and health policy [27]. Limiting the harm caused by new infections such as COVID-19 demands far greater attention to non-communicable diseases and socioeconomic inequality than has hitherto been admitted.

Parks and Thalheimer extend the idea of cascading and compound stressors to include not only the pandemic, but also climate change and migration, and their interactional impact on mental health (see Figure 1.1 [28]).

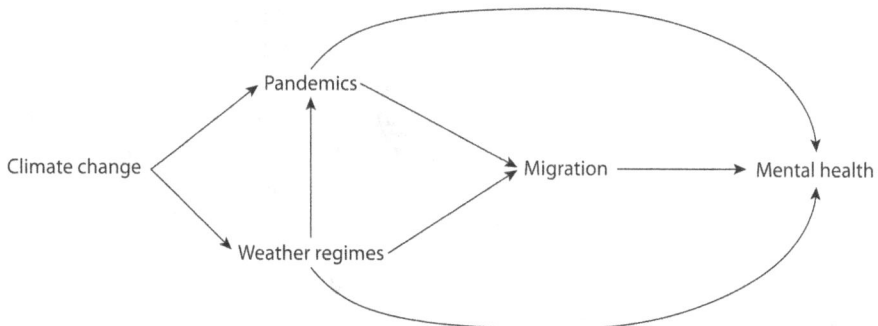

FIGURE 1.1 Cascading and compound stressors.

They propose a formalised framework of how climate change, migration, and COVID-19 impact each other and mental health. They argue that the compounding effect of multiple serious and simultaneous natural hazards along with COVID-19 and other pandemics, in tandem with the impact of a changing climate on those migrating and the communities they arrive at, puts strain on a society's ability to cope with the negative impacts of compounding vulnerabilities.

We would extend this model further to include the impact of socio-economic and gender inequalities that lead to disparities and discriminations, as well as the impact of geopolitical conflicts affecting peace and security within countries or regions. But our analysis and conclusions are the same: all of these multi-dimensional factors act – and interact – to adversely affect the mental health of individuals and communities.

The intense and prolonged nature of the pandemic has put significant strain on healthcare professionals, including family physicians and primary care practitioners. Burnout and secondary traumatic stress (compassion fatigue) are serious concerns and even prior to the COVID-19 pandemic several concerns have been published [29, 30]. Physicians may experience emotional exhaustion, decreased empathy, and a sense of being overwhelmed due to the high demands and emotional toll of caring for patients during the pandemic. Supporting the mental well-being of healthcare professionals will be crucial to ensure their own health and the quality of care they provide as a recent opinion to European Commission has clearly revealed [31].

IMPACT OF COMBINED CRISES
Impact on Mamadou

In the case of 23-year-old Mamadou, who we introduced at the beginning of this chapter, we can see how all the elements of this syndemic interact to adversely affect his health. Climate change in his home country has destroyed his family's economic prospects and has led to political instability and military rule. He saw no option but to leave in hope of a better life, which so far has not materialised. Instead, his hazardous migration journey has left him with severe mental health problems (distress, sleep disturbance, and possible hallucinations), while his breathing and muscle problems are likely related to long-COVID. Social isolation and perceived discrimination have been included in the psychosocial determinants of cardiovascular disease, while among migrants the impact of social isolation either on psychosocial responses (e.g., depression and quality of life) or on health-related behaviours (i.e., self-care), or clinical responses (e.g., cognitive function and health service use) is currently discussed [32].

Impact on primary care professionals

These multi-dimensional factors also impact on the mental health of primary care professionals. We may experience stress and burnout from the increased workload and emotional tolls as climate change or geopolitical conflict impact patients like Mamadou. Working with migrant populations adds additional challenges, including language barriers, cultural differences, and ethical dilemmas, which can contribute to mental health disorders. The combined impact of these stressors can lead to higher levels of burnout, anxiety, depression, and other mental health disorders, affecting our ability to provide adequate care.

In addition, witnessing the physical and psychological impacts of climate change, pandemics, geopolitical threats, and forced migration on patients, including injuries, illnesses, and trauma, can have an emotional toll on primary care professionals. We may experience grief, frustration, and helplessness, contributing to burnout and compassion fatigue issues that have been extensively studied before and during the COVID-19 pandemic. Primary care professionals who are environmentally conscious may experience distress and anxiety about the long-term implications of climate change on public health.

Continually witnessing the distress and suffering of migrants can impact the mental well-being of primary care professionals, leading to symptoms of vicarious trauma and compassion fatigue. The migrant crisis also introduces cultural and language challenges, as evidenced by specific European collaborative projects, including RESTORE and EUR-HUMAN. This European experience shows that primary care professionals providing care to migrants may face challenges related to language barriers, cultural differences, and diverse healthcare beliefs and practices. These challenges can increase communication, diagnosis, and treatment complexity, potentially contributing to frustration and stress.

Ethical and moral dilemmas may also be introduced by the migrant crisis. Primary care professionals may grapple with ethical and moral dilemmas when addressing the healthcare needs of migrants, particularly in situations where resources are limited or legal and social barriers impede access to care. These dilemmas can contribute to moral distress and psychological strain.

Primary care professionals may personally experience the consequences of climate change and migration crises, such as being affected by extreme weather events or having their communities impacted by forced displacement. These personal experiences can further contribute to our mental health challenges and influence our ability to provide care effectively.

Those of us who have been privileged to experience life in western Europe during past 50 years can no longer delude ourselves that we live in an orderly, comfortable, predictable world. Certainty has been replaced by contingency. We now live in deeply troubled times, with severe threats facing us in irrevocable climate change, pandemic infections, and cataclysmic conflict. We can no longer dismiss these problems as the preserve of others. They are at our own doorstep. They directly affect our own lives, and the lives of those we love. We must acknowledge the existential unease [33] that this reality generates not only in our patients but also in ourselves.

Challenges for the healthcare system and services

The pandemic has highlighted existing disparities in mental health access and outcomes. Family physicians and primary care practitioners encounter populations with higher vulnerability to mental health challenges, including marginalised communities, low-income individuals, and those with limited access to resources. Addressing these disparities and providing equitable mental health care will require targeted efforts, community partnerships, and culturally sensitive approaches.

Telepsychiatry and digital mental health solutions have become increasingly important during the pandemic, allowing for remote consultations and interventions. Frontline physicians, as above, may need to adapt and incorporate these technologies into their practice to provide mental health support to patients. However, challenges such as ensuring technological access, maintaining patient privacy, and adapting to virtual care delivery methods have been discussed widely in the literature and they deserve further attention.

As mental health needs increase, effective collaboration and coordination between primary care practitioners, mental health specialists, and community support services become paramount. Establishing referral networks, improving communication channels, and developing care pathways to ensure seamless transitions between primary care and specialized mental health care will be crucial for providing comprehensive and integrated healthcare, and enhancing the healthcare system's resilience.

Communal threats and responses

These perspectives on emerging mental health challenges mean we must set aside deeply entrenched individualistic perspectives on the causes and management of emotional distress. They force us to acknowledge the profound existential threats facing all members of all societies, including those in the global North who have – until recently – considered themselves immune to catastrophe. They call on us to develop communal understandings and collective responses to human suffering.

The Cross-Cultural RE-ORDER study, involving interviews with family physicians and people of Vietnamese and East Timorese origin in Melbourne Australia, posed a central dilemma: How to integrate experiences grounded in one social context within the matrices provided by another [34]? We identified a *tremendous collision* between migrants, whose experience was framed by patterns of alienation and traumatized self-identity, and family physicians, who interpreted distress as technical problems of practice.

Migrants saw their suffering as related to family disintegration, marital breakdown, intergenerational conflict, immigration issues, and cultural distance:

> *Oh, my first impression was that it was so cold... It was cold. From Malaysia where it was hot, we had on only light clothing. So it was terribly cold. It was on a Saturday that we arrived; there was no one in the city. ... I thought how come there were no people in this country. The streets were deserted. I thought now I was in another country, and I did not know English, I did not know how I would start a new life. That was my continuing worry.*

Faced with such communal and structural accounts of suffering, the family physicians opted to defend and draw on an individualised notion of depression in performing their work and accounting for the distress presented to them:

> *I think most people understand sadness, and quite a lot of people understand depression as a condition that can require treatment; but in some cultures, they don't understand it as a condition that requires treatment.*

In this context, the diagnosis of depression was not a clinical entity, but a mechanism of decoupling: replacing loss with illness, it individualised previously social problems. In doing so, family physicians were effectively distancing themselves from the reality of the suffering being presented.

Instead, we need to extend our gaze and acknowledge the wider determinants of our patients' emotional distress. We should be aware of the causes of mental illness, not just its symptoms and the consequences.

At the individual level, we can usefully move beyond a simplistic reliance on diagnosis, and adopt the practice of making a *formulation* to guide our care of patients [35]. Detection and diagnosis of a mental health problem on the basis of symptoms, function, and duration should be accompanied by a clinical review – or formulation – for each person which takes into account their values and preferences, their life stories, and the circumstances (e.g., their migration story, the effects of poverty or extreme weather) in which they find themselves.

We can also bear witness to our patients' suffering in the face of overwhelming life experiences and difficulties. We can take heart from Virgil's epic story of Aeneas as a refugee, driven far from home by the vicious ravages of the Trojan War, and his phrase *'sunt lacrimae rerum'* [36]. In Latin, *rerum* is the genitive of *res* (things) and can be understood in both objective and subjective terms. So this phrase has been translated as either 'there are tears for things', or else 'there are tears of things'. The first, objective version indicates the burdens we have to bear, the frailty of human existence, the 'shit life syndrome' so many patients experience. The second, subjective version indicates that things feel sorrow for our suffering – that in some sense the universe feels our pain.

Virgil is fully aware of the ambiguity and wishes for us to understand both meanings at the same time. So does Seamus Heaney, who translates the phrase as, 'There are tears at the heart of things' [37]. At that moment when I experience and express compassion for the suffering of the person in the room with me, both senses of *sunt lacrimae rerum* are present. My patient can express pain, distress, and suffering, knowing that – from me – he finds understanding, compassion, and safety. My consulting room has become, at least momentarily, a sanctuary [38].

There is emerging evidence of the beneficial effects of clinical compassion in primary care [39] supporting migrants, isolated people, and other vulnerable groups [40–42]. Patients' perceptions of family doctors' empathy are key to enablement, which leads to improvement in symptom severity and related well-being [43]. Antidepressant medications are associated with better outcomes when provided by supportive and empathic family doctors [44].

There is also a need to strengthen communal responses to support individuals and families who struggle from socioeconomic inequalities.

However, we cannot expect to tackle these immense problems alone; that would be a recipe for burnout, exhaustion, and compassion fatigue. As family doctors, we must make common cause with health and social care colleagues, community actors, and policymakers to provide effective and compassionate care where it is most urgently needed.

NEW AND EMERGING SOLUTIONS

We offer three case studies drawn from our experience of local and international collaborative research projects, to show how these new and emerging mental health challenges may be addressed by new and emerging collaborative solutions. The first is an example of family doctors developing collaborative links with other stakeholders in their local communities. The second and third are examples of family doctors working collectively across different countries.

Improving access to mental health in primary care (AMP)

In order to increase access to high-quality primary mental health care for underserved groups, the AMP partnership created a model of care with three discrete but interacting elements: community engagement, primary care training, and tailored psychosocial interventions (see Figure 1.2).

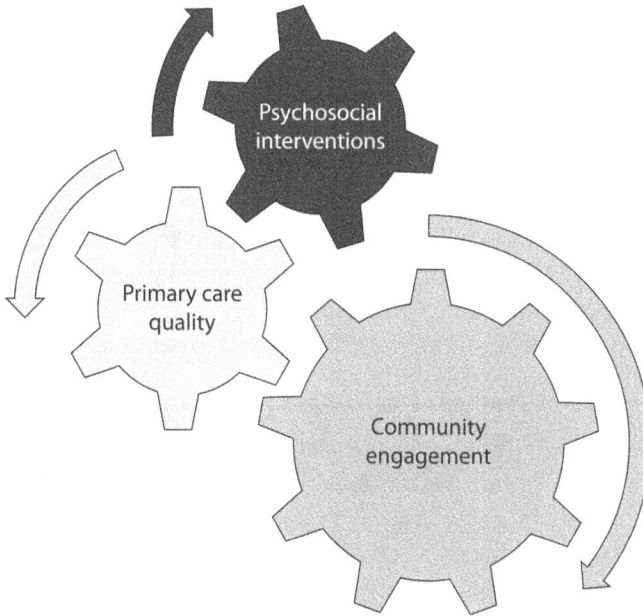

FIGURE 1.2 The AMP Partnership Model.

Community engagement included the identification of 'community champions' and the creation of community focus groups to negotiate the aims and agenda of the intervention with local people, agencies, and wider stakeholders, and agree an action plan. The primary care element includes active linking between family doctors and relevant local organizations and resources.

The model was implemented in four underserved localities in North-West England, focusing on older people and minority ethnic populations. Using a quasi-experimental design with no-intervention comparators, we gathered a combination of quantitative and qualitative information.

We found evidence that the three elements of the AMP model did interact effectively. Access to the psychosocial interventions was related to the presence of the community engagement and the primary care training elements. Referrals to the psychosocial interventions were associated with community engagement, while recruitment was associated with primary care training. Qualitative data suggested that the mechanisms underlying these associations were increased awareness and sense of agency. The quality of primary mental health care was enhanced by information gained from our community mapping activities, and by the offer of access to the psychosocial interventions. We also found that participation in the psychosocial interventions led to increased community engagement [45].

Investing in workforce and training initiatives

EUR-HUMAN

The ongoing refugee crisis has revealed the need for enhancing primary health care (PHC) professionals' skills and training. The aim of the European Refugees–Human Movement and Advisory Network (EUR-HUMAN) was to strengthen PHC professionals in European countries in the provision of high-quality care for refugees and migrants by offering concise modular training based on the needs of the refugees and PHC professionals [42].

We developed, piloted, and evaluated an online capacity-building course of eight stand-alone modules containing information about acute health issues of refugees, legal issues, provider–patient communication and cultural aspects of health and illness, mental health, sexual and reproductive health, child health, chronic diseases, health promotion, and disease prevention. The English course template was translated into seven languages and adapted to the local contexts of six countries. Pre- and post-completion knowledge tests were administered to effectively assess the progress and knowledge increase of participants so as to issue Continuing Medical Education (CME) certificates. An online evaluation survey post-completion was used to assess the acceptability and practicability of the course from the participant perspective.

A total of 390 participants registered for the online course in six countries, almost half (48%) of them medical doctors. The mean time for completion was 10.77 hours. The modules on acute health needs, legal issues (both 44%), and provider–patient communication/cultural issues (53%) were found particularly important for the daily practice. A majority expressed a will to promote the online course among their peers.

We consider this course to be a promising learning tool for PHC professionals, with the potential to empower them in their work with refugees and other migrants [46].

ADVOCACY project

The World Health Organization (WHO) recognizes the essential role of mental health in achieving health for all; its mental health action plan calls for more effective leadership for mental health and the provision of community-based, integrated care [47]. However, integrating mental health care into primary care is a challenging, transformational change that requires more than clinical knowledge. It depends on strong advocacy, leadership, and change management: skills that can be learned [48].

The Farley Health Policy Center located in Colorado, USA partnered with the World Organization of Family Doctors to develop and pilot a global curriculum to enable learners to lead practice transformation and be empowered with policy-influencing skills to advocate for their patients, to promote and enhance primary care mental health. We recruited 12 young family doctors, of whom 7 were women and 10 were from low- and middle-income countries.

The learners were divided into two learning cohorts. Sessions were facilitated by two leaders and supported by four mentors. The educational content was delivered twice (to accommodate differing time zones) in six 90-minute monthly virtual sessions. The learners also developed individual projects to undertake in their own locality, with support and guidance from their cohort's mentors and facilitators, and feedback from other learners.

Despite initiation in the midst of the COVID-19 pandemic, this pilot project was successfully implemented with remarkable commitment of participants. The structure and operations of the programme were confirmed to be feasible. The imbedded evaluation provided important insights for improvement and affirmation that the programme was relevant, desired, and acceptable in different country environments. The learners formed their own community, finding their heterogeneity enriching. Several learners, already in positions of influence, recognized their ability to advocate for policy change [49].

RECOMMENDATIONS

In conclusion, we offer six recommendations to family doctors and primary health practitioners when addressing these new and emerging challenges.

1. *Stay informed*: Keep up to date with (reputable) information on the social, environmental, and political stressors that affect you and your patients.
2. *Use formulations*: Do not simply make a diagnosis. Take account of your patients' values and preferences, their life stories, and their personal circumstances before agreeing on the best options for their care.
3. *Bear witness to suffering*: Compassion makes a difference.
4. *Form alliances and take collective action*: We cannot achieve systemic change on our own. Find and work with local and international partners.
5. *Take care of your own mental health*: Follow the five principles of self-care:
   - *Preparation*: Maintain optimum sleep, diet, and exercise, pursue hobbies and accept vulnerability in all spheres.
   - *Protection*: Monitor your own physical and emotional health, staying attuned to early warning signs such as substance misuse.
   - *Professionalism*: Limit external information to a few reliable sources, stay abreast of important news and medical updates, and dispel misinformation.
   - *Promotion*: Be a role model of staff, patients, and students, keeping calm, looking after others, and using self-compassion.
   - *Pathways*: Ensure you see your own family doctor as needed [50].
6. *Retain hope*: It is 'an important tool to protect well-being and foster activism in the face of adversity' [51]. Hopelessness leads to despair and inertia. Hope enables us to seek, test, and deliver on solutions.

REFERENCES

1. United Nations Website. https://news.un.org/en/news/topic/peace-and-security. accessed 30 July 2024
2. https://www.ipcc.ch/report/ar6/syr/downloads/report/IPCC_AR6_SYR_SPM.pdf accessed 13 July 2023
3. Richards C, Gauch H, Allwood J. International risk of food insecurity and mass mortality in a runaway global warming scenario. Futures. 150;2023:103173. https://doi.org/10.1016/j.futures.2023.103173
4. Wellcome Trust. https://wellcome.org/news/explained-how-climate-change-affects-mental-health. accessed 13 July 2023
5. Burke M, González F, Baylis, P. Heft-Neal S, Baysan C, Basu S, et al. Higher temperatures increase suicide rates in the United States and Mexico. Nature Clim Change. 2018;8:723–729.
6. Romanello M, McGushin A, Di Napoli C, Green C, Kennard H, Lampard P, et al. The 2021 report of the Lancet Countdown on health and climate change: code red for a healthy future. Lancet. 2021 Oct 30;398(10311):1619–1662.
7. Newbury JB, Stewart R, Fisher HL, Beevers S, Dajnak D, Broadbent M, et al. Association between air pollution exposure and mental health service use among individuals with first presentations of psychotic and mood disorders: retrospective cohort study. Br J Psychiatry. 2021 Dec;219(6):678–685.
8. Hickman C, Marks E, Pihkala P, Lewandowski RE, Mayall EE, Wray B, et al. Climate anxiety in children and young people and their beliefs about government responses to climate change: a global survey. Lancet Planet Health. 2021 Dec;5(12):e863–e873.
9. Ogunbode C, Pallesen S, Böhm G, Doran R, Bhullar N, Aquino S, et al. Negative emotions about climate change are related to insomnia symptoms and mental health: cross-sectional evidence from 25 countries. Curr Psychol. 2023;42:845–854.
10. Lawrance EL, Jennings N, Kioupi V, Thompson R, Diffey J, Vercammen A. Psychological responses, mental health, and sense of agency for the dual challenges of climate change and the COVID-19 pandemic in young people in the UK: an online survey study. Lancet Planet Health. 2022 Sep;6(9):e726–e738.
11. World Health Organization. https://www.who.int/publications/i/item/9789240004528. 2020 accessed 13 July 2023
12. Atwoli L, Muhia J, Merali Z. Mental health and climate change in Africa. BJPsych International. 2022;19(4):86–89.
13. Huntington M, Gavagan T. Disaster medicine training in family medicine: a review of the evidence. Fam Med. 2011;43(1):13–20.
14. Cunsolo Willox A, Harper S, Ford J, Edge V, Landman K, Houle K, et al. Climate change and mental health: an exploratory case study from Rigolet, Nunatsiavut, Canada. Climatic Change. 2013;121:255–270.
15. World Health Organization. https://www.who.int/news-room/feature-stories/detail/the-impact-of-covid-19-on-mental-health-cannot-be-made-light-of#:~:text=A%20great%20number%20of%20people,affected%20much%20more%20than%20others. 2022 accessed 13 July 2023
16. WONCA COVID and Mental Health Webinar. https://www.youtube.com/watch?v=QDX2AFKtcgw accessed 13 July 2023
17. World Health Organization (Europe). https://apps.who.int/iris/bitstream/handle/10665/342932/WHO-EURO-2021-2845-42603-59267-eng.pdf. 2020 accessed 13 July 2023
18. Guardian Newspaper. https://www.theguardian.com/society/2023/jun/21/health-workers-suicidal-thoughts. 2023 accessed 13 July 2023
19. Ahrendt D, Mascherini M, Nivakoski S, Sandor E. Living, working and COVID-19: mental health and trust decline across EU as pandemic enters another year. 2021. Dublin:

Eurofound. https://www.eurofound.europa.eu/publications/report/2021/living-working-and-covid-19-update-april-2021-mental-health-and-trust-decline-across-eu-as-pandemic

20. Shi LS, Xu RH, Xia Y, Chen DX, Wang D. The impact of COVID-19-related work stress on the mental health of primary healthcare workers: the mediating effects of social support and resilience. Front Psychol. 2022 Jan 21;12:800183. https://doi.org/10.3389/fpsyg.2021.800183

21. Evered JA, Castellanos MEP, Dowrick A, Camargo Goncalves Germani AC, Rai T, et al. Talking about inequities: a comparative analysis of COVID-19 narratives in the UK, US, and Brazil. SSM Qual Res Health. 2023 Jun;3:100277

22. https://www.redcross.org.uk/about-us/what-we-do/how-we-support-refugees/find-out-about-refugees accessed 21 August 2023

23. Close C, Kouvonen A, Bosqui T, Patel K, O'Reilly D, Donnelly M. The mental health and wellbeing of first generation migrants: a systematic-narrative review of reviews. Global Health. 2016;12(1):47.

24. Priebe S, Giacco D, El-Nagib R. Public Health Aspects of Mental Health Among Migrants and Refugees: A Review of the Evidence on Mental Health Care for Refugees, Asylum Seekers and Irregular Migrants in the WHO European Region. Copenhagen: WHO Regional Office for Europe; 2016. Report No.: 9789289051651.

25. Bogic M, Njoku A, Priebe S. Long-term mental health of war-refugees: a systematic literature review. BMC Int Health Hum Rights. 2015;15:29.

26. George U, Thomson MS, Chaze F, Guruge S. Immigrant mental health, a public health issue: looking back and moving forward. Int J Environ Res Public Health. 2015;12(10):13624–13648.

27. Singer M, Bulled N, Ostrach B, Mendenhall E. Syndemics and the biosocial conception of health. Lancet. 2017 Mar 4;389(10072):941–950. https://doi.org/10.1016/S0140-6736(17)30003-X

28. Parks R, Thalheimer L. IOM UN Migration. The hidden burden of pandemics, climate change and migration on mental health. https://environmentalmigration.iom.int/blogs/hidden-burden-pandemics-climate-change-and-migration-mental-health accessed on 7th July

29. Soler JK, Yaman H, Esteva M, et al. Burnout in European family doctors: the EGPRN study. Fam Pract. 2008 Aug;25(4):245–265.

30. Msaouel P, Keramaris NC, Tasoulis A, Kolokythas D, Syrmos N, Pararas N, et al. Burnout and training satisfaction of medical residents in Greece: will the European Work Time Directive make a difference? Hum Resour Health. 2010 Jul 1;8:16.

31. Barros P, Rogers H, Zalatel J, de Maeseneer J, Garcia-Altes A, Kringos D, et al. Expert panel on effective ways of investing in health. Opinion on supporting mental health of health workforce and other essential workers. 2021. https://health.ec.europa.eu/system/files/2021-10/028_mental-health_workforce_en_0.pdf

32. Iovino P, Vellone E, Cedrone N, Riegel B. A middle-range theory of social isolation in chronic illness. Int J Environ Res Public Health. 2023 Mar 10;20(6):4940.

33. Tomasdottir MO, Sigurdsson JA, Petursson H, Kirkengen AL, Ivar Lund Nilsen T, et al. Does 'existential unease' predict adult multimorbidity? Analytical cohort study on embodiment based on the Norwegian HUNT population. BMJ Open. 2016 Nov 16;6(11):e012602.

34. Kokanovic R, May C, Dowrick C, Furler J, Newton D, Gunn J. Negotiations of distress between East Timorese and Vietnamese refugees and their family doctors in Melbourne. Sociol Health Illn. 2010;32:511–527.

35. Herrman H, Patel V, Kieling C, Berk M, Buchweitz C, Cuijpers P, et al. Time for united action on depression: a Lancet-World Psychiatric Association Commission. Lancet. 2022 Mar 5;399(10328):957–1022.

36. P Vergilius Maro, *Aeneid*, 29-19 BC. Book 1, lines 461-3

37. Seamus Heaney, *Virgil's Poetic Influence*, an essay broadcast on BBC Radio 3 as part of the Greek and Latin Voices series, 2008 July 15 (23:00).

38. Dowrick C. Suffering and hope: Helen Lester Memorial Lecture 2016. BJGP Open. 2017 Feb 15;1(1):bjgpopen17X100605.

39. Jani BD, Blane DN, Mercer SW. The role of empathy in therapy and the physician-patient relationship. Forsch Komplementmed. 2012;19:252–257.

40. Shea S, Lionis C. Restoring humanity in health care through the art of compassion: an issue for the teaching and research agenda in rural health care. Rural Remote Health. 2010 Oct–Dec;10(4):1679.

41. Lionis C, Petelos E, Mechili EA, Sifaki-Pistolla D, Chatzea VE, Angelaki A, et al. Assessing refugee healthcare needs in Europe and implementing educational interventions in primary care: a focus on methods. BMC Int Health Hum Rights. 2018 Feb 8;18(1):11

42. van Loenen T, van den Muijsenbergh M, Hofmeester M, Dowrick C, van Ginneken N, Mechili EA, et al. Primary care for refugees and newly arrived migrants in Europe: a qualitative study on health needs, barriers and wishes. Eur J Public Health. 2018 Feb 1;28(1):82–87.

43. Mercer SW, Higgins M, Bikker AM, Fitzpatrick B, McConnachie A, Lloyd SM, et al. General practitioners' empathy and health outcomes: a prospective observational study of consultations in areas of high and low deprivation. Ann Fam Med. 2016 Mar;14(2):117–124.

44. van Os TW, van den Brink RH, Tiemens BG, Jenner JA, van der Meer K, Ormel J. Communicative skills of general practitioners augment the effectiveness of guideline-based depression treatment. J Affect Disord. 2005;84:43–51.

45. Dowrick C, Bower P, Chew-Graham C, Lovell K, Edwards S, Lamb J, et al. Evaluating a complex model designed to increase access to high quality primary mental health care for under-served groups: a multi-method study. BMC Health Serv Res. 2016 Feb 17;16:58.

46. Jirovsky E, Hoffmann K, Mayrhuber EA, Mechili EA, Angelaki A, Sifaki-Pistolla D, et al. Development and evaluation of a web-based capacity building course in the EUR-HUMAN project to support primary health care professionals in the provision of high-quality care for refugees and migrants. Glob Health Action. 2018;11(1):1547080.

47. Global Mental Health Action Network. Global Mental Health Advocacy Road Map 2020–2021. https://unitedgmh.org/sites/default/files/2021-01/Roadmap_v5.pdf. 2021 accessed 1 September 2023

48. Koch U, Bitton A, Landon BE, Phillips RS. Transforming primary care practice and education: lessons from 6 academic learning collaboratives. J Ambul Care Manag. 2017;40(2):125–138.

49. Amor SH, Daniels-Williamson T, Fraser-Barclay K, Dowrick C, Gilchrist EC, Gold S, et al. Advocacy training for young family doctors in primary mental health care: a report and global call to action. BJGP Open. 2022 Mar 22;6(1):BJGPO.2021.0163.

50. Benson J, Sexton R, Dowrick C, Lionis C, Ferreira Veloso Gomes J, Bakola M, et al. Staying psychologically safe as a doctor during the COVID-19 pandemic. Fam Med Community Health. 2022 Jan;10(1):e001553.

51. Frumkin H, Cook S, Dobson J, Abbasi K. Mobilising hope to overcome climate despair. BMJ 2022;379:o2411

CHAPTER 2

Long-COVID and mental health

Characterization, treatment options, implications for service delivery and recommendations for delivery

Heather L. Rogers and Christos Lionis

INTRODUCTION

Paul, a 45-year-old man, works in a small factory in an urban area of Greece. He has four children and faces significant challenges in effectively managing family responsibilities. Paul is a smoker, has elevated blood pressure, and often experiences low moods and emotional distress. Following a COVID-19 infection, Paul returns to his work and even four weeks after the infection, he continues to struggle with persistent symptoms, including shortness of breath, fatigue, and a lingering cough. These health issues have negatively impacted his ability to perform at work, placing him at risk of losing his job. As his depressive symptoms have worsened over time, Paul decided to consult his personal doctors, seeking advice and support to address his physical and mental health concerns.

'Long-COVID' refers to a grouping of signs, symptoms, and conditions that develop or persist in individuals with a history of probable or confirmed SARS-COVID-19 infection. Long-COVID is not one condition. It represents many potentially overlapping entities, likely with different biological causes and sets of risk factors and outcomes [1]. Some of the terms synonymous with Long-COVID include post-COVID syndrome, post-acute COVID-19, chronic

COVID-19, long-term effects of COVID, and long-haul COVID. In general, what they have in common is that the signs, symptoms, and conditions (a) are present four or more weeks after infection, (b) may affect multiple body systems, and (c) may relapse, remit and/or progress or worsen over time [2]. The clinical case definition from the World Health Organization (WHO) in October 2021 indicated that 'Post-COVID Condition' typically occurs three months after symptomatic COVID-19, with symptoms that last for at least two months and cannot be explained by an alternative diagnosis [3]. In October 2022, the International Classification of Diseases, Tenth Edition (ICD-10-CM) assigned U09.9 to 'Post-COVID Condition', unspecified [4]. Typical physical symptoms of 'Post-COVID Condition' include fatigue, muscle or joint pain, shortness of breath, and impaired sleep [5]. According to an Advisory by the Substance Abuse and Mental Health Services Administration (SAMHSA) of the United States published in June 2023 [6], the mental health conditions associated with Long-COVID include, but are not limited to, depression, anxiety, psychosis, obsessive compulsive disorder, and post-traumatic stress disorder.

LONG-COVID AND MENTAL HEALTH

This chapter focuses on the intersection of Long-COVID and mental health in adults. Little is known about this area in children at the time of writing (Fall 2023), although study protocols are ongoing (e.g., the CLoCk study by Stephenson and colleagues) [7]. Long-term outcomes remain uncertain. Based on a recently published review [8], Long-COVID in children can lead to school absenteeism, social withdrawal, and psychological distress, potentially affecting cognitive development. Similarly, research on mental health and its associated symptoms and conditions as related to Long-COVID in adults is constantly evolving. The relationship is complex and bidirectional. For instance, one study followed individuals who did not report SARS-CoV-2 infection at baseline in April 2020 for one year. Of those who reported a positive SARS-CoV-2 test result during follow-up, self-reported depression, anxiety, perceived stress, loneliness, and worry about COVID-19 were prospectively associated with a 1.3- to 1.5-fold increased risk of self-reported post-COVID-19 conditions, as well as increased risk of daily life impairment related to post-COVID-19 conditions [9]. Another study, Taquet and colleagues [10], followed patients diagnosed with COVID-19 between January and August 2020 for 90 days. They found that people without prior mental health conditions were at increased risk of a first psychiatric diagnosis compared with six other health events (influenza, other respiratory tract infections, skin infection, cholelithiasis, urolithiasis, fracture of a large bone) [10]. The numerous potential mechanisms have been hypothesized and are still being investigated, for example by Monje and Iwasaki [11].

A meta-analysis by Premraj and colleagues [12] used the National Institute for Healthcare Excellence (NICE) definition of post-COVID-19 syndrome (symptoms that develop or persist ≥3 months after the onset of COVID-19) and examined mental health symptoms. This work provides some benchmark for the prevalence of anxiety and depressive symptoms in Long-COVID. Despite the methodological limitations of existing research (including small sample sizes, heterogeneity in defining the case group and difficulties identifying a control group), they estimated that approximately one-quarter of Long-COVID sufferers experience anxiety symptoms and one out of ten experience depressive symptoms. Sub-group analyses provided further insight. When they compared patients hospitalized for acute COVID-19 to non-hospitalized patients, hospitalized patients had *reduced* frequency of anxiety and depression at three or more months post-infection. Yet, a *higher* prevalence of anxiety and depression was identified in cohorts with >20% of patients admitted to the ICU during acute COVID-19 vs. cohorts with <20% of ICU admission [12].

Van der Feltz-Cornelis and colleagues [13] conducted a systematic review and meta-analysis to estimate the prevalence of mental health conditions and brain fog. They found that, in 17 studies of 41,249 individuals with Long COVID, the combined prevalence was 20.4% and lower among those previously hospitalized than in community-managed individuals. At 12 months, the combined prevalence was 27.4% [14].

Gallegos and colleagues [14] question the assumption that the most persistent symptoms affecting mental health are a direct consequence of COVID-19 infections. Although many studies have focused on documenting these symptoms, few have examined the extent to which they are specifically caused by the virus. Despite a widely accepted causal relationship, as of writing, the evidence is not yet sufficiently clear. It is crucial to recognize the specific physiological and neurobiological impacts of COVID-19 on health, which has led to a renewed focus on mental health conditions. This shift may mark the beginning of a broader integration of mental health into the healthcare system, and into primary care specifically.

TREATMENT AND INTERVENTION APPROACHES FOR LONG-COVID MENTAL HEALTH SYMPTOMS

Unsurprisingly, the evidence base for treatment and intervention for Long-COVID is generally weak. The WHO living guideline for the management of COVID-19 has a large section dedicated to the rehabilitation of adults with Post-COVID-19 Condition [15]. Mental health is addressed as Topic 11 and is described in more detail in the WHO guidelines. Currently, evidence for effective ways to address mental health in the context of Long-COVID is scarce and generally relies heavily on how anxiety and depression are effectively managed in other chronic conditions. A systematic review of registered trials examining interventions for mental health, cognition, and psychological well-being in patients with Long-COVID was published by Hawke and colleagues [15] and thus there is reason to be optimistic that more solid conclusions with respect to effective treatment and intervention approaches will be forthcoming from this research.

The WHO living guideline [15] suggests the use of psychological support for the clinical rehabilitation management of anxiety and depression in adults with Post-COVID-19 Condition. Effective treatments for anxiety and depression in general include interpersonal therapy, cognitive-behavioural therapy (CBT), behaviour activation, and problem-solving counseling. Preliminary evidence suggests that CBT programs may be effective in patients with prior COVID-19 [16], including video-based formats of CBT [17].

The WHO living guideline [15] also suggests physical exercise training when the individual does not have Post-Exertional Symptom Exacerbation (PESE). Physical exercise training that includes aerobic exercise has been shown to reduce depression and anxiety symptoms in patients with a respiratory condition and those with an immediate history of COVID-19. A symptom-titrated exercise program is recommended. In this approach, physical activity is continuously monitored and adjusted according to the presenting symptoms aiming to achieve sustainable symptom stabilization. Both structured and unstructured exercise programs have been found to lead to subjective improvements in quality of life. A 2019 Cochrane Review [18] indicated that CBT and co-intervention such as aerobic exercise may reduce depressive symptoms more than aerobic exercise alone in individuals with chronic pulmonary obstructive disease.

The WHO living guideline [15] cites evidence of small improvements in mental health within breast cancer patients to suggest mindfulness-based approaches (e.g., mindfulness mediation or mindfulness-based stress reduction) using a structured individual or group program. The guideline also highlights the usefulness of encouraging peer support. Individuals suffering from Long-COVID indicate that peer group support is helpful, validating, and alleviating distress. Social media and online face-to-face support groups have been identified as a valuable way to share experiences, knowledge, and resources with others in a similar situation. Individuals reported being reassured that they were not alone in their struggle with long-term symptoms [19].

A scoping review by Al-Jabr and colleagues [20] identified studies reporting on a variety of interventions to support mental health among people with Long-COVID. They report that although all those studied reported positive changes, methodological limitations (e.g., being case studies) indicate that caution is warranted. There is a clear need for more research to be conducted to identify the impact of interventions on mental health of people with Long-COVID, especially with respect to the role of primary care services, as discussed in the next section.

SERVICE DELIVERY – IMPLICATIONS FOR PRIMARY CARE

Primary care faces numerous challenges when it comes to managing Long-COVID-19. There is evidence that Long-COVID increases healthcare utilization. In a recent 2024 study, Lin and colleagues [21] reported that people with Long-COVID were more likely to use healthcare resources (OR: 8.29, 95% CI: 7.74–8.87) and have 49% more healthcare utilization (RR: 1.49, 95% CI: 1.48–1.51) in the 12 months post-diagnosis than a comparator group without the diagnosis. This clearly invites a strong primary care contribution.

In this regard, it is crucial to first recognize, and then to treat, this condition. Landhuis [22] reports in the *Journal of the American Medical Association*, a relevant clinical case that addresses this issue. In general, patients often feel unheard, while physicians also feel frustrated due to the lack of resources, information, and time to attend to Long-COVID patients. This underscores the need for additional training for primary care providers to meet the diverse needs of patients with Long-COVID. It is also essential to adapt the healthcare system in ways that address these barriers, for instance allowing longer visit times for patients presenting with Long-COVID and/or working in multidisciplinary treatment teams. Although multidisciplinary models are predominantly found in academic centers and large cities across the United States, most care for Post-Acute Sequelae of SARS-CoV-2 is provided by primary care providers. Barshikar and colleagues [23] describe how the primary care model relates to Post-COVID Condition. Specifically, primary care providers screen patients presenting with symptoms related to Long-COVID. Through established algorithms and a consensus-based approach, healthcare systems that include primary care can manage symptoms, incorporate various therapy disciplines, and facilitate referrals. Furthermore, home care and virtual visits via primary care staff could have the potential to improve access to care in underserved populations. For these reasons, and many more, primary care seems to be the most appropriate place to meet the needs of Long-COVID patients.

In the United States, List and Long [24] describe community-based primary care management of long-COVID. This involves primary care staff responding quickly to, and meeting, the needs of individual and community COVID-19 survivors, which includes addressing potential complications and the mental health impact of the pandemic. They recommend that, in areas heavily impacted by the COVID-19 pandemic, primary care practices should proactively reach out to patients who may have been hospitalized with severe illness to support their recovery course.

Primary care is accustomed to adapting to new contexts. Long-COVID brings new challenges and experiences. Rotar Pavlic and colleagues [25] interviewed Slovenian primary care physicians and reported that the problems they faced can be divided into two groups: either biological health-related or psychological. They advocate for the importance of good communication and increased trust between physicians and patients as critical for an integrated model of managing Long-COVID.

It is important for the primary care provider to be familiar with the full range of Long-COVID symptoms [22], otherwise misdiagnosis can result [27]. Primary care staff must take great care in their communication to acknowledge and validate the patient's complaints. If the patient perceives that the care provider thinks that they are exaggerating or somatizing psychological symptoms, shame and embarrassment may result. The patient may then not seek out further medical treatment.

Primary care becomes especially critical with respect to vulnerable populations and health inequities. It is well documented that acute COVID-19 is associated with racial disparities [28] and vulnerable individuals facing post-acute and Long-COVID may have little or no health insurance coverage. Furthermore, Berger and colleagues [29] identify another obstacle that disproportionately affects vulnerable individuals with Long-COVID: the disabling symptoms of this illness, which hinder the sufferer's ability to work and contribute to increased dependency. Therefore, they argue that 'primary care providers are uniquely positioned to provide and coordinate care for vulnerable patients with long-COVID' [29]. To meet this challenge, primary care providers should be well trained and equipped with the skills to conduct 'an assessment of the multisystem disorder and make judicious referrals to cardiology, respiratory, neurological, mental health, or other specialist colleagues as needed' [29]. The implication is that professional training, including medical student curriculums and continuing education courses, should be adapted accordingly.

It implies significant changes in the delivery of healthcare services and underscores the need for integrated approaches. Collaboration between primary care, mental health professionals, and specialists is crucial to addressing the multifaceted needs of Long-COVID patients.

KEY POINTS

- Long-COVID represents several potentially overlapping entities likely with different biological causes and sets of risk factors and outcomes.
- The relationship between mental health and its associated symptoms and conditions as related to Long-COVID is complex and bidirectional. Research is still evolving.
- The evidence-base for specific mental health treatment approaches in the context of Long-COVID is still developing. Psychological support in the form of CBT and physical exercise training are promising interventions.
- The implications for primary care service delivery include ensuring that primary care providers are well trained and equipped with the skills to conduct an assessment of the multisystem disorder and make

judicious referrals, including evaluation of mental health and well-being and appropriate follow-up care.
- Given the uncertainties around Long-COVID and the lack of definitive curative therapies, primary care providers should implement person-centred care to address the whole person, including social determinants of health, and consider using a trauma-informed treatment approach to benefit their patients.

RECOMMENDATIONS FOR PRIMARY CARE PROVIDERS

The COVID-19 pandemic and its effects, including Long-COVID, has placed the focus back on the importance of mental health. Primary care, as the first point of contact with healthcare, plays an essential role in differential diagnosis, monitoring mental health, and determining the most appropriate therapeutic approach. Greenhalgh and colleagues [26] highlight role of generalist primary care physicians to include: 'hearing and affirming the patient's story; excluding red flag conditions or symptoms; educating and explaining; arranging multidisciplinary team input (eg, community physiotherapy); managing co-morbidities; organizing investigations and referrals as indicated; working with the patient to set goals and monitor progress against them, including, where appropriate, self-monitoring of symptoms; recommending or prescribing symptomatic remedies; and providing sickness certification.' (p. 714). Adopting a person-centred approach becomes the cornerstone of Long-COVID care delivery, in which the patient as a person is holistically addressed. For instance, Essien [30] recommends addressing reported symptoms with empathy and compassion, and taking into account the patient's psychosocial characteristics – including social determinants of health and psychological characteristics – which affect mental health. Symptoms, including mental health as a direct cause of Long-COVID or consequence of Long-COVID, must be managed in the consultation or through referrals to qualified specialists from other disciplines (e.g., social work, psychology, psychiatry, physical therapy, pharmacology). Furthermore, she also encourages strategies to engage the patient in shared decision-making and empowering them to manage their care. Landhuis [22] also focuses on the primary care provider's attitude toward the patient with Long-COVID using a whole-person approach. Her four basic guidelines for primary care providers are: (1) believe the patient, (2) go beyond the symptoms, (3) address fatigue, and (4) look for familiar, overlapping conditions.

Greenhalgh and colleagues [31], in their Practice Pointer for the *British Medical Journal* (BMJ), remind healthcare providers of the uncertainties around Long-COVID and the lack of definitive curative therapies. In addition to the recommendations discussed in the prior paragraph, they also advocate listening and validating the patient's narrative, identifying, and acting on 'red flag' symptoms, setting realistic goals for recovery, and providing certification so that the patient can request time off (sick leave) from work. From a research perspective, it is also critical to document appropriately. They emphasize the importance of coding the diagnosis of Long-COVID [4] correctly in the electronic medical record, which would facilitate researchers' ability to fill gaps in current knowledge on this evolving condition [32].

In conclusion, Long-COVID for patients may be associated with trauma of a life-altering chronic illness. Therefore, primary care providers are encouraged to take a trauma-informed treatment approach when working with these patients [33]. A trauma-informed approach involves numerous important aspects: emphasizes safety, trustworthiness, and transparency; focuses on collaboration and mutuality; empowers the individual; acknowledges cultural, historical, and gender issues; and may include peer support [34]. Additional training in implementation of trauma-focused primary care [35] for primary care providers may be valuable.

FURTHER READING AND e-RESOURCES

- https://www.who.int/news-room/fact-sheets/detail/post-covid-19-condition-(long-COVID)
  - Fact sheet on Post COVID-19 condition (long-COVID) published in early 2025.
- https://www.who.int/teams/health-care-readiness/post-covid-19-condition
  - Resources from the WHO regarding Post COVID-19 conditions, including a WHO Guidelines Development Group for clinical management, clinical case definitions, and a publication on Living Guidance for Clinical Management with recommendations for rebabilitation of adults with post COVID-19 condition.
- https://library.samhsa.gov/sites/default/files/pep23-06-05-007.pdf
  - The SAMHSA published this Advisory in Summer 2023 on the identification and management of mental health symptoms and conditions associated with Long-COVID.
- http://eppi.ioe.ac.uk/cms/Projects/DepartmentofHealthandSocialCare/Publishedreviews/COVID-19Livingsystematicmapoftheevidence/tabid/3765/Default.aspx
  - Living map of the evidence on COVID-19 created by the Evidence for Policy and Practice Information Centre at University College London. There is a section on Long-COVID and another section on quarterly scoping of the Long-COVID literature (at the time of writing).
- https://www.bmj.com/content/378/bmj-2022-072117
  - BMJ Practice Pointer article from 2022 which includes resources for patients and an infographic for primary care providers.
- https://bestpractice.bmj.com/topics/en-gb/3000327
  - BMJ Best Practice site on Long-COVID that is regularly reviewed and updated as needed. It includes information on the definition, history and exam, and diagnostic interventions. There is a section for a treatment algorithm as well.

REFERENCES

1. Ely EW, Brown LM, Fineberg HV; National Academies of Sciences, Engineering, and Medicine Committee on Examining the Working Definition for Long COVID. Long-COVID Defined. N Engl J Med. 2024 Nov 7;391(18):1746–1753. doi: 10.1056/NEJMsb2408466. https://www.nejm.org/doi/full/10.1056/NEJMsb2408466

2. Soriano JB, Murthy S, Marshall JC, Relan P, Diaz JV; WHO Clinical Case Definition Working Group on Post-COVID-19 Condition. A clinical case definition of post-COVID-19 condition by a Delphi consensus. Lancet Infect Dis. 2022 Apr;22(4):e102–e107. doi: 10.1016/S1473-3099(21)00703-9. https://doi.org/10.1016/S1473-3099(21)00703-9

3. World Health Organization. A clinical case definition of post COVID-19 condition. WHO. 2021. Available from: https://www.who.int/publications/i/item/WHO-2019-nCoV-Post_COVID-19_condition-Clinical_case_definition-2021.1

4. ICD-10-CM Code. ICD-10-CM Code U09.9. Available from: https://www.icd10data.com/ICD10CM/Codes/U00-U85/U00-U49/U09-/U09.9

5. World Health Organization. Clinical management of COVID-19. WHO. 2023. Available from: https://www.who.int/publications/i/item/WHO-2019-nCoV-clinical-2023.2

6. Substance Abuse and Mental Health Services Administration. SAMHSA Advisory: Identification and Management of Mental Health Symptoms and Conditions Associated with Long-COVID. SAMHSA. 2023. Available from: https://library.samhsa.gov/sites/default/files/pep23-06-05-007.pdf

7. Stephenson T, Shafran R, De Stavola B, Rojas N, Aiano F, Amin-Chowdhury Z, McOwat K, Simmons R, Zavala M, Consortium C, Ladhani SN. CLoCk Consortium members. Long COVID and the mental and physical health of children and young people: national matched cohort study protocol (the CLoCk study). BMJ Open. 2021 Aug 26;11(8):e052838. https://doi.org/10.1136/bmjopen-2021-052838

8. Basaca D-G, Jugănaru I, Belei O, Nicoară D-M, Asproniu R, Stoicescu ER, Mărginean O. Long COVID in children and adolescents: mechanisms, symptoms, and long-term impact on health—a comprehensive review. J. Clin Med. 2025;14:378. https://doi.org/10.3390/jcm14020378

9. Wang S, Quan L, Chavarro JE, Slopen N, Kubzansky LD, Koenen KC, Kang JH, Weisskopf MG, Branch-Elliman W, Roberts AL. Associations of depression, anxiety, worry, perceived stress, and loneliness prior to infection with risk of post–COVID-19 conditions. JAMA Psychiatry. 2022;79(11):1081–1091. https://doi.org/10.1001/jamapsychiatry.2022.2640

10. Taquet M, Luciano S, Geddes JR, Harrison PJ. Bidirectional associations between COVID-19 and psychiatric disorder: retrospective cohort studies of 62,354 COVID-19 cases in the USA. Lancet Psychiatry. 2021;8(2):130–140. https://doi.org/10.1016/S2215-0366(20)30462-4

11. Monje M, Iwasaki A. The neurobiology of long COVID. Neuron. 2022 Nov 2;110(21):3484–3496. https://doi.org/10.1016/j.neuron.2022.10.006

12. Premraj L, Kannapadi NV, Briggs J, Seal SM, Battaglini D, Fanning J, Suen J, Robba C, Fraser J, Cho SM. Mid and long-term neurological and neuropsychiatric manifestations of post-COVID-19 syndrome: a meta-analysis. J Neurol Sci. 2022 Mar 15;434:120162. https://doi.org/10.1016/j.jns.2022.120162

13. Van der Feltz-Cornelis C, Turk F, Sweetman J, Khunti K, Gabbay M, Shepherd J, Montgomery H, Strain WD, Lip GYH, Wootton D, Watkins CL, Cuthbertson DJ, Williams N, Banerjee A. Prevalence of mental health conditions and brain fog in people with long COVID: A systematic review and meta-analysis. Gen Hosp Psychiatry. 2024 May-Jun;88:10–22. doi: 10.1016/j.genhosppsych.2024.02.009.

14. Gallegos M, Portillo N, Martino P, Cervigni M. Long COVID-19: rethinking mental health. Clinics (Sao Paulo). 2022 Jun 13;77:100067. https://doi.org/10.1016/j. clinsp.2022.100067

15. Hawke LD, Nguyen ATP, Ski CF, Thompson DR, Ma C, Castle D. Interventions for mental health, cognition, and psychological wellbeing in long COVID: a systematic review of registered trials. Psychol Med. 2022 Oct;52(13):2426–2440. https://doi. org/10.1017/S0033291722002203

16. Li J, Li X, Jiang J, Xu X, Wu J, Xu Y. The effect of cognitive behavioral therapy on depression, anxiety, and stress in patients with COVID-19: a randomized controlled trial. Front Psychiatry. 2020;11:596.

17. Shabahang R, Bagheri Sheykhangafshe F, Dadras M, Seyed Noori SZ. Effectiveness of video-based cognitive-behavioral intervention on health anxiety and anxiety sensitivity of individuals with high levels of COVID-19 anxiety. J Clin Psychol. 2021;13(2):33–44.

18. Pollok J, van Agteren JE, Esterman AJ, Carson-Chahhoud KV. Psychological therapies for the treatment of depression in chronic obstructive pulmonary disease. Cochrane Database Syst Rev. 2019 Mar 6;3(3). https://doi.org/10.1002/14651858. CD012347

19. Macpherson K, Cooper K, Harbour J, Mahal D, Miller C, Nairn M. Experiences of living with long COVID and of accessing healthcare services: a qualitative systematic review. BMJ Open. 2022;12(1):e050979. https://doi.org/10.1136/bmjopen-2022-068481.

20. Al-Jabr H, Hawke LD, Thompson DR, Clifton A, Shenton M, Castle DJ, Ski CF. Interventions to support mental health in people with long COVID: a scoping review. BMC Public Health. 2023 Jun 20;23(1):1186. https://doi.org/10.1186/ s12889-023-16079-8

21. Lin LY, Henderson AD, Carlile O, Dillingham I, Butler-Cole BFC, Marks M, Briggs A, Jit M, Tomlinson LA, Bates C, Parry J, Bacon SCJ, Goldacre B, Mehrkar A, MacKenna B; OpenSAFELY Collaborative; Eggo RM, Herrett E. Healthcare utilisation in people with long COVID: an OpenSAFELY cohort study. BMC Med. 2024;22:255. https://doi. org/10.1186/s12916-024-03477-x

22. Landhuis EW. How primary care physicians can recognize and treat long COVID. JAMA. 2023 May 23;329(20):1727–1729. https://doi.org/10.1001/jama.2023.6604

23. Barshikar S, Laguerre M, Gordon P, Lopez M. Integrated care models for long coronavirus disease. Phys Med Rehabil Clin N Am. 2023 Aug;34(3):689–700. https:// doi.org/10.1016/j.pmr.2023.03.007

24. List JM, Long TG. Community-based primary care management of 'Long COVID': A center of excellence model at NYC Health+ hospitals. Am J Med. 2021 Oct;134(10): 1232–1235. https://doi.org/10.1016/j.amjmed.2021.05.029

25. Rotar Pavlic D, Maksuti A, Mihevc M, Munda A, Medija K, Strauch V. Long COVID as a never-ending puzzle: the experience of primary care physicians. A qualitative interview study. BJGP Open. 2023 Dec 19;7(4). https://doi.org/10.3399/ BJGPO.2023.0074

26. Greenhalgh T, Sivan M, Perlowski A, Nikolich JŽ. Long COVID: a clinical update. Lancet. 2024 Aug 17;404(10453):707–724. doi: 10.1016/S0140-6736(24)01136-X.

27. Byrne EA. Understanding long COVID: nosology, social attitudes and stigma. Brain Behav Immun. 2022;99:17–24. https://doi.org/10.1016/j.bbi.2021.09.012

28. Kumar S, Kumar P, Kodidela S, Duhart B, Cernasev A, Nookala A, Kumar A, Singh UP, Bissler J. Racial health disparity and COVID-19. J Neuroimmune Pharmacol. 2021 Dec;16(4):729–742. https://doi.org/10.1007/s11481-021-10014-7

29. Berger Z, Altiery DE Jesus V, Assoumou SA, Greenhalgh T. Long COVID and health inequities: the role of primary care. Milbank Q. 2021 Jun;99(2):519–541. https://doi.org/10.1111/1468-0009.12505

30. Essien E, AcademyHealth. Long COVID and care delivery challenge: the role of health services research. 2023. Available from: https://academyhealth.org/blog/2023-01/long-covid-and-care-delivery-challenge-role-health-services-research

31. Greenhalgh T, Sivan M, Delaney B, Evans R, Milne R. Long COVID—an update for primary care. BMJ. 2022;378:e072117. https://doi.org/10.1136/bmj-2022-072117

32. Henderson AD, Butler-Cole BF, Tazare J, Tomlinson LA, Marks M, Jit M, Briggs A, Lin LY, Carlile O, Bates C, Parry J, Bacon SC, Dillingham I, Dennison WA, Costello RE, Wei Y, Walker AJ, Hulme W, Goldacre B, Mehrkar A, MacKenna B; OpenSAFELY Collaborative; Herrett E, Eggo RM. Clinical coding of long COVID in primary care 2020-2023 in a cohort of 19 million adults: an OpenSAFELY analysis. EClinicalMedicine. 2024 May 17;72:102638. https://doi.org/10.1016/j.eclinm.2024.102638

33. Griffin G. Defining trauma and a trauma-informed COVID-19 response. Psychol Trauma. 2020;12(S). https://doi.org/10.1037/tra0000828

34. Substance Abuse and Mental Health Services Administration (SAMHSA). SAMHSA's concept of trauma and guidance for a trauma-informed approach. HHS Publication No. (SMA). 2014;. 14–4884. Available from: https://library.samhsa.gov/sites/default/files/sma14-4884.pdf

35. Hamberger LK, Barry C, Franco Z. Implementing trauma-informed care in primary medical settings: evidence-based rationale and approaches. J Aggress Maltreat Trauma. 2019;28(4):425–444. https://doi.org/10.1080/10926771.2019.1572399

CHAPTER 3

Mental health in the post-COVID period

A global health challenge

Marilena Anastasakis, Ferdinando Petrazzuoli, and Christos Lionis

INTRODUCTION

Petros is a 24-year-old man originating from a rural area of Greece. Upon receiving his first degree, he continued his studies in a master's program at a regional university. There are financial restrictions in his family: his father, a 68-year-old farmer, has advanced lung cancer and is unable to work; however, he has to contribute to his son's tuition fees. Petros also works nightshifts at a restaurant to cover some of his and his family's expenses. He presents at your practice in spring of 2024 with persistent anxiety, restlessness, and difficulty sleeping. These began approximately six months after recovering from a mild COVID-19 infection and one month after his registration in his Master's. He reports excessive worry about his career, financial stability, the possibility of reinfection, and the health of his father. His symptoms have worsened over time, significantly impairing his work performance and daily functioning. He has no prior mental health diagnoses and no visible medical conditions. He had contracted mild COVID-19 again in 2022, recovering at home. No family history of mental illness is reported, although his father presents depressive symptoms due to his severe illness. Petros lives alone in a rented apartment next to his workplace, which lost several clients during the pandemic. He reports isolation habits as a residual of the pandemic, as well as a means to protect his father's health. He looks well groomed, but anxious. His mood denotes constant worry due to fears about his future. He has mild

DOI: 10.1201/9781003473947-5

attention deficits and obvious suffering from his condition. He recognizes
the excess of his symptoms but struggles to control them.

Global health is a multidisciplinary field focused on improving health and achieving equity in health for all people worldwide. It addresses transnational health issues, determinants, and solutions through collaborative, interdisciplinary actions [1]. Mental health is now recognized as a vital component of overall well-being and development. Mental health conditions, including depression, anxiety, and substance use disorders, are leading causes of disability globally [2]. Despite this, access to mental health care remains limited, especially in low- and middle-income countries [3, 4]. Integrating mental health into global health is essential for achieving sustainable, inclusive, and holistic health outcomes for all people worldwide.

The COVID-19 pandemic caused widespread disruptions, with isolation, uncertainty, and economic strain deeply affecting global mental health [5]. Prolonged lockdowns and social distancing measures led to loneliness and disconnection, particularly among young people, who also faced school closures, disrupted routines, and limited access to social support [6]. Economic instability further intensified stress, as many families experienced job losses and financial insecurity. Young individuals reported heightened fears about their future, academic setbacks, and health anxieties, both for themselves and loved ones. Healthcare systems, strained by the pandemic, fell short in addressing the unmet needs of adolescents and young people, while the essential healthcare and social workforce was faced with an unprecedented demand for services with minimal administrative or managerial support [7]. These conditions fostered a surge in anxiety, depression, and emotional distress, leaving lasting psychological impacts on a generation already navigating a complex world [8].

Two well-recognized concepts that appeared more and more frequently during the COVID-19 pandemic were vulnerability and suffering. The last one was particularly absent from the conversations between physicians and patients prior to the pandemic [9]. Another word that was sharply introduced into the scientific vocabulary was that of resilience. Petros, in our case, is visibly suffering due to his personal and family circumstances. He is young and vulnerable; he is not able to cope with his current situation and has no resilience mechanisms. He is expecting much from his family physician who, like most healthcare professionals, is charged with reducing their patients' suffering and inability to cope with post-COVID life, not only through medical treatments but also through psychological support.

In the general population, the COVID-19 pandemic exacerbated or triggered a range of mental health issues, including anxiety disorders, depression, post-traumatic stress disorder (PTSD), substance abuse, and burnout [5, 10, 11]. These conditions significantly impacted global health, contributing to increased disability, reduced quality of life, and heightened suicide risk. Healthcare services faced overwhelming demand for mental health support, often without adequate infrastructure or workforce capacity. In many regions, mental health services were disrupted or deprioritized [12]. Economically, untreated mental health conditions reduced productivity, increased absenteeism, and strained social support systems [13]. The global economy continues to bear the cost of this mental health crisis, with long-term implications for development.

Additionally, the global mental health crisis in the post-COVID period is unfolding alongside other major global challenges, such as climate change, armed conflicts, and forced displacement. These co-existing crises have intensified psychological distress, especially in vulnerable populations [14, 15]. Climate-related disasters and environmental degradation contribute to eco-anxiety and trauma, while wars and political instability displace millions, exposing them to chronic stress, loss, and uncertainty. Combined with the lingering impacts of the pandemic, these factors have overwhelmed health systems and deepened inequalities in mental health care. Addressing mental health now requires a holistic global response that acknowledges the interconnected nature of these overlapping crises.

It is evident that the COVID-19 pandemic left a profound and lasting impact on global mental health, triggering a surge in anxiety, depression, and stress-related disorders across all age groups and regions. As the world transitions into the post-COVID period, mental health has emerged as a critical global health challenge, revealing deep-seated inequalities in access to care and support. This chapter explores the multifaceted consequences of the pandemic on psychological well-being, the social and economic determinants exacerbating mental distress, and the urgent need for integrated, inclusive mental health strategies to address this silent yet escalating crisis in global public health.

MENTAL HEALTH DURING THE COVID-19 PANDEMIC
Emerging stressors – Social isolation, economic anxiety, and health-related fears

The COVID-19 pandemic introduced multiple key stressors that significantly impacted global mental health. Social isolation and loneliness surged as lockdowns and physical distancing disrupted daily life and human connection. A global survey found that over 40% of adults in the United States reported increased feelings of loneliness [16]. Economic anxiety also intensified, with a documented loss of 255 million full-time jobs worldwide in 2020 alone, leading to widespread financial insecurity [17]. Health-related fears – such as fear of infection, hospitalization, or death – were pervasive. A study estimated a 25% global increase in anxiety and depression during the first year of the pandemic [5]. These stressors, often occurring simultaneously, created a compounded burden on mental health, disproportionately affecting low-income groups, youth, and frontline workers, and exposing critical gaps in mental health infrastructure across high- and low-income countries alike. Social isolation, economic anxiety, and health-related fears are also present in Petros' case.

Impact on mental health figures of the general population

During the COVID-19 pandemic, rates of anxiety, depression, PTSD, and substance abuse significantly increased worldwide. It is estimated that anxiety disorders rose by 25.6%, while major depressive disorders increased by 28% globally [5]. In the United States, 31% of adults experienced symptoms of anxiety or depression, and 13% started or increased substance use [18]. PTSD symptoms were notably high among frontline workers and COVID-19 survivors, with studies showing prevalence rates ranging from 20% to 30% [19]. These trends strained healthcare systems and underscored urgent mental health needs.

Beyond mental health diagnoses and conditions, suffering itself is a broader experience. Epstein (2017) emphasizes that suffering extends beyond disease, encompassing psychological, existential, spiritual, financial, and social dimensions [9]. In our clinical case, Petros' suffering reflects all of these, and his primary care provider is called upon to support and empower him through this complexity.

Impact on mental health of primary care providers in rural settings

The COVID-19 pandemic has undeniably impacted the physical and mental health of all population groups. However, healthcare workers appear to be one of the most vulnerable groups due to the high risk of infection, increased work stress, and fear of spreading the infection to their families [20–22]. However, prior to the crisis, the well-being of this group was already of concern [23]. Primary care providers (PCPs) in rural areas often carry a heavy burden of care, including mental health, leading to burnout, and reduced capacity. In a European study conducted in 33 countries, a significant difference between mixed urban–rural practices compared to those in cities and suburbs was observed. GPs working with more vulnerable patient populations were at higher risk of distress. In particular, those having an average or more than average proportion of patients with financial difficulties were associated with higher distress [23]. Significant differences in well-being scores were noted between countries. Collaboration from other practices and perception of having adequate governmental support were significant protective factors for distress.

Burnout, which was common among family physicians even before the pandemic [24], reached epidemic levels among healthcare providers well before this health crisis, and is the most extreme form of a lack of well-being. Symptoms presented by healthcare workers include depression, depersonalization, emotional exhaustion, a sense of reduced personal accomplishment, anxiety, stress, and cognitive and social problems. These symptoms, when they occur, have a direct impact not only on the physician but also on the patient [20]. Studies have shown that among physicians who report experiencing at least some signs of burnout, family medicine and emergency medicine physicians are among those at highest risk [25].

Family physicians working in larger practices, usually located in an urban area, are more satisfied and have fewer burnout symptoms than those working in single-handed, usually rural practices [23, 26]. One's perception of having adequate governmental support, experiencing collaboration from practices in the neighborhood, and having enough protected time to review guidelines and scientific literature are significant protective factors for distress [23, 26].

Impact on women's mental health – Violence against women in rural settings

A UK study assessing the decline in mental health of the population after the onset of the COVID-19 pandemic found a significant age–gender gradient, with the decline being more than twice as large for women as for men and young females suffering particularly badly. This might relate to younger women's perceived loss of social interaction or more uncertain work conditions during the pandemic [27]. Research shows a gender-differentiated impact of COVID-19 on women, with women experiencing a more pronounced decline in mental well-being compared to men [28, 29]. This was attributed in part to increased care responsibilities and changes in employment status, where women faced higher job loss rates than men.

Women living in urban areas generally reported a higher perceived negative impact on mental health compared to women in rural areas or in small-/ medium-sized towns [30, 31]. Studies conducted in different countries have confirmed that caring for children during the pandemic had a negative impact on mental health and this may be due to the fact that in many households, lockdowns, and curfews meant more childcare for women [32, 33].

The perceived increase in violence against women during the pandemic influenced the impact of lockdowns and curfews on mental health, especially in rural areas [31]. In any case, this issue was present before the pandemic in 2015. Edwards conducted a review on the urban/rural IPV divide which found that rural women experienced more chronic and severe intimate partner violence (IPV) and had more severe psychosocial and physical health outcomes, including increased PTSD, due to the lack of IPV-related services [34].

In our clinical case, Petros' mother is a key person experiencing increased vulnerability that should not be overlooked during Petros' therapeutic process. She is caring for her severely ill husband while also worrying about Petros' condition. This added emotional burden may lead to increased suffering, anxiety, and possibly depressive symptoms, highlighting the need for family-oriented support from PCPs.

Impact on other vulnerable populations – Children, elderly, people with severe mental illness, socioeconomically deprived groups

The disruption of schooling, socialization, and routine exacerbated mental health issues in children [35]. The World Health Organization (WHO) reported that one in five children experienced symptoms of anxiety and depression during the pandemic [36]. The closure of schools, limited access to mental health resources, and uncertainty about the future led to increases in behavioural problems, academic struggles, and emotional distress. Children from low-income families were particularly vulnerable, facing additional stressors like food insecurity and lack of access to digital learning resources [37].

The elderly experienced significant mental health challenges due to prolonged isolation, fear of illness, and limited social interaction during lockdowns. Studies indicate that social isolation among the elderly increased significantly during the pandemic, contributing to heightened rates of anxiety, depression, and cognitive decline [38, 39]. Studies have found that older adults reported feelings of loneliness present worsened mental health outcomes [40, 41].

Individuals with severe mental illness faced challenges due to interrupted mental health services, medication shortages, and fears about COVID-19 transmission in healthcare settings. Individuals with schizophrenia, bipolar disorder, and other severe conditions saw worsened symptoms and disruptions in care during the pandemic, leading to a spike in psychiatric hospital admissions [42].

Low-income and marginalized communities were hit hardest by economic insecurity, inadequate healthcare, and poor living conditions. These groups experienced elevated levels of anxiety, depression, and substance use. A study found that during the pandemic, the odds of individuals with household incomes less than USD 19,999 of experiencing depression symptoms increased 2.4 times compared to those with incomes of USD75,000 or more [43].

In our clinical case, all the above are features of Petros' family and should be taken into consideration by the physician: financial restrictions, advanced age, severe illness in his father, and potentially poor access to community and primary healthcare services.

Long-term implications – Long-COVID, suicide rates, domestic violence, mental health crises

The long-term implications of the COVID-19 pandemic extend far beyond the initial health crisis, with lasting effects on mental health, social dynamics, and overall well-being. Two of the most pressing concerns in the post-pandemic period are Long-COVID and the surge in suicide rates, domestic violence, and mental health crises [44–46].

Long-COVID refers to the prolonged symptoms experienced by individuals after recovering from the acute phase of the virus. These symptoms, as also presented in detail in Chapter 2 of this book, include fatigue, brain fog, muscle pain, and anxiety, and they often lead to significant disruptions in daily life. In a nationwide population cohort of Scottish adults, 64.5% of individuals reported at least one COVID-19 symptom six months following SARS-CoV-2 infection [44]. This condition has placed a strain on healthcare systems, with individuals needing long-term care, rehabilitation, and mental health support. Furthermore, the stress and uncertainty surrounding Long-COVID have contributed to the rise of anxiety and depression, as individuals struggle to cope with ongoing symptoms and a diminished quality of life [47].

Simultaneously, the pandemic has exacerbated existing mental health issues, leading to alarming increases in suicide rates and domestic violence. Evidence suggests that an upward trend of suicidal ideation and suicide attempts was observed during the COVID-19 pandemic [48]. Social isolation, financial stress, and the constant uncertainty about health have contributed to rising suicide rates, especially among vulnerable populations such as the elderly and young adults. In the United States, suicide rates significantly increased between 2020 and 2021 for males aged 15–24, 25–44, 65–74, and 75 and over [49]. In our clinical case, the provider caring for Petros, along with managing various clinical responsibilities and completing a mental health assessment, should also prioritize the critical task of exploring the presence of suicidal ideation.

Domestic violence incidents also surged during lockdowns. The United Nations (UN) reported that one in three women globally experienced violence during the pandemic, with calls to domestic violence helplines increasing [50]. The lockdowns, financial pressures, and heightened stress have made it harder for victims to escape abusive situations, exacerbating the crisis.

The overall increase in mental health crises is staggering. The consequences are felt across healthcare systems, economies, and societies, highlighting the need for comprehensive mental health support and policy responses to address the long-term toll of the pandemic.

MENTAL HEALTH IN THE POST-COVID PERIOD

In the post-COVID-19 era, global mental health has faced significant challenges, with anxiety, depression, and other disorders affecting populations worldwide [51]. A study revealed that approximately 50% of individuals globally are likely to develop a mental disorder by age 75, a substantial increase from previous estimates [52]. Young people have been particularly affected, with a UN report highlighting a decline in youth happiness in countries like the United States, United Kingdom, and Australia attributed to factors such as social media influence and reduced physical activity [53].

The impact of global disparities in mental health outcomes in the post-COVID period

In the post-COVID period, inequalities in access to mental health care have widened, disproportionately affecting low-income countries compared to high-income countries. The pandemic exacerbated pre-existing disparities, with low-income countries struggling to provide adequate mental health services due to limited resources, insufficient infrastructure, and a shortage of trained professionals. According to the WHO, over 70% of people with mental health conditions in low-income countries receive no treatment, compared to only 35% in high-income countries [54].

In contrast, high-income countries have better access to mental health care, with more established support systems, funding, and telehealth services. The WHO noted that high-income countries invested more in mental health during the pandemic, leveraging digital health solutions and providing financial support for mental health programs [54]. However, even in high-income countries, mental health care systems have been overwhelmed, highlighting that the gap between the rich and poor in terms of mental health care availability is a global issue [55, 56].

Marginalized groups, particularly racial and ethnic minorities, faced greater exposure to COVID-19 risks due to systemic healthcare inequities and frontline employment [57–59]. Additionally, the disruption of social support networks, compounded by lockdowns and social distancing, further isolated these communities, worsening mental health outcomes. The lack of culturally competent mental health services in many regions exacerbated these issues, as vulnerable populations often lack access to appropriate care. In particular, studies have demonstrated that marginalized populations experienced a higher incidence of mental health challenges during the pandemic [60]. For instance, a US study found substantial disparities for marginalized identities by gender, sexual orientation, and disability status with each ethnicity sub-sample showing a unique pattern of relationships between COVID-19 risk and mental health symptoms [61].

Frontline healthcare practitioners have experienced unprecedented levels of stress and burnout in the post-COVID period, significantly impacting their well-being and the quality of patient care [62]. A study in Western Greece found that over 40% of healthcare workers reported high levels of emotional exhaustion, with nurses and paramedics being particularly affected [63]. In the United States, a survey revealed that 62% of healthcare workers experienced negative mental health impacts due to pandemic-related stress, with 55% feeling burned out [64].

ADDRESSING THE GLOBAL MENTAL HEALTH CHALLENGE
Barriers toward a global mental health strategy

Addressing the global mental health challenge requires a multifaceted approach, focused on improving access to care, increasing funding, and reducing stigma. The WHO highlights that approximately one in four people will experience a mental health disorder in their lifetime, yet mental health services are severely underfunded, particularly in low-income countries [65]. This shortage limits access to essential care, especially in rural and underserved areas [66].

To address these gaps, governments must significantly increase funding for mental health services. A key focus should be on integrating mental health into primary care, as suggested by the WHO's Mental Health Gap Action Programme (mhGAP), which promotes the delivery of basic mental health services by primary care workers. Additionally, enhancing mental health education and reducing stigma is crucial for encouraging people to seek help [67].

The identification of barriers impeding a global mental health strategy is essential to addressing the increasing burden of mental health disorders worldwide. One significant barrier is the global shortage of mental health professionals and services. According to the WHO, there is a critical shortage of mental health services, with an estimated global average of only 0.64 community-based mental health facilities per 100,000 population. There is extreme variation between income groups, with 0.11 facilities per 100,000 population in low-income countries and 5.1 facilities per 100,000 population in high-income countries [68]. This shortage limits access to care, particularly in rural and underserved areas, where mental health services are often unavailable.

Another major barrier is insufficient funding for mental health services. The WHO estimates that, globally, less than 1% of health budgets are allocated to mental health [68]. In low-income countries, this figure can be even lower. For example, in Africa, the average mental health expenditure is less than US$0.50 per capita, while in high-income countries, it exceeds US$50 [66]. This severe underfunding hampers the development of adequate mental health infrastructure, such as hospitals, community clinics, and trained professionals, which is crucial for effective care delivery.

Moreover, gaps in mental health infrastructure are widespread, particularly in rural and isolated areas. Many countries, especially in sub-Saharan Africa and Southeast Asia, lack sufficient mental health facilities and services integrated into primary healthcare systems, contributing to an environment where individuals with mental health issues do not receive timely or adequate care [67].

The COVID-19 pandemic has significantly strained healthcare systems globally, leading to increased mental health inequalities. The surge in physical health cases during the pandemic, coupled with limited healthcare resources, has created competition between physical and mental health services. According to the WHO, the pandemic resulted in a 25% increase in anxiety and depression globally [69]. However, mental health services have struggled to keep up with this demand. Many health systems were overwhelmed by COVID-19 cases, leading to the diversion of resources away from mental health care, which was often considered less urgent.

This competition for resources has resulted in underfunding for mental health promotion. The WHO reports that in many countries, mental health budgets were either reduced or remained stagnant during the pandemic, despite the rising need for services. Moreover, the delayed provision of mental health services has worsened long-term outcomes, creating deeper mental health inequalities, particularly for vulnerable populations such as healthcare workers, children, and those with pre-existing conditions.

In addition to these factors, the stigma surrounding mental health in many cultures, alongside the lack of standardized mental health policies and data collection, impedes global progress [70, 71]. A coordinated and well-funded global strategy, focusing on equitable resource allocation, policy development, and infrastructure strengthening and training of mental health professionals is essential to overcoming these barriers and improving mental health care worldwide. Collaboration between governments, international organizations, and communities is vital to creating a more equitable and effective mental health system worldwide.

The need for global health policy and international collaboration

A global healthcare policy focused on mental health is essential to address the escalating burden of mental health disorders worldwide. Mental health issues have become a leading cause of disability, yet there is a significant gap in mental health resources and support. To address this, international collaboration is crucial. A global health coalition, comprising the WHO, the UN, the European Commission (EC), and other international health organizations, can play a pivotal role in promoting mental health globally.

The WHO's leadership in mental health, through initiatives like the Mental Health Action Plan, is a critical starting point [68]. However, its efforts need stronger backing from global entities such as the UN, which can advocate for mental health as a fundamental human right, and the EC, which can help align policies across European nations. Collaborative strategies should aim to increase funding, standardize mental health care policies, and integrate mental health services into primary care systems globally.

A global health coalition could facilitate cross-border research, share best practices, and ensure mental health issues are prioritized on the international health agenda. Additionally, global coordination is vital to reduce mental health disparities, especially in low-income countries, where services are often inadequate. Only through collaboration and robust policy development can a comprehensive global strategy for mental health be achieved [72].

Innovative practices are essential to address the global mental health challenge, particularly in low-resource settings. One promising approach is the integration of mental health into primary care. The WHO mhGAP promotes training primary healthcare providers to offer basic mental health care, which has been shown to improve access and reduce stigma [73]. This model has been successfully implemented in countries like India and Uganda, where community health workers provide mental health support in rural areas, reaching populations otherwise underserved.

Telemedicine is another innovative practice gaining traction. Digital platforms and mobile applications offer remote mental health services, providing therapy and counseling to individuals in regions with limited access to trained professionals. The use of apps like *Headspace* and *Woebot* has been shown to be effective in reducing symptoms of anxiety and depression, especially during the COVID-19 pandemic [74].

BUILDING INTEGRATED AND RESILIENT MENTAL HEALTH SYSTEMS
Why invest in mental health services

Building integrated and resilient mental health systems requires a holistic approach that combines mental health with general healthcare. The WHO advocates for integrating mental health into primary care, which improves access and reduces stigma [75]. In high-income countries, integrated systems have led to improved outcomes, such as in the United Kingdom's National Health System (NHS), where mental health services are embedded in general practices [76]. Additionally, resilient systems should be adaptable to crises, like the COVID-19 pandemic, where telemedicine became essential in maintaining care [77]. Strong policy frameworks and adequate funding are key for sustainability.

National healthcare strategies must focus on sustainable mental health policies, adequate funding, and the training of healthcare providers. For example, the United Kingdom's 'Five Year Forward View for Mental Health' strategy significantly increased funding for mental health services, resulting in improvements in access and quality in care [76]. These strategies must be adapted to national contexts, ensuring comprehensive mental health services that are equitable, accessible, and culturally sensitive.

Petros' case, in our clinical scenario, highlights the evolving role of family physicians and PCPs in an era where mental health problems are increasing. It underscores the importance of providing strong support and guidance to the younger generation to alleviate suffering and reduce symptoms, through the integration of mental health into primary care, enhancing professional skills, and strengthening health systems.

Advocacy for increased global funding and resources for mental health

Investing in mental health services is critical to addressing the growing global burden of mental health disorders. The WHO estimates that nearly one in four people will experience a mental health condition at some point in their lives [78]. Despite this, mental health receives a disproportionately low share of global health funding [66]. This lack of investment has resulted in insufficient infrastructure, a shortage of trained professionals, and limited access to care, particularly in low- and middle-income countries.

Increased global funding and resources are essential to meet the rising demand for mental health services. Already, since 2016, the WHO has called for countries to allocate at least 5% of their health budgets to mental health [79]. This investment would help improve mental health services, ensure accessibility, and reduce stigma. Additionally, investing in mental health can yield significant economic returns. Studies show that every US$1 invested in mental health treatment can result in a return of US$4 in improved health and productivity [80].

Global advocacy efforts must also focus on policy development, integrating mental health into primary care systems, and fostering international collaboration to share resources and knowledge. A comprehensive, well-funded approach to mental health will enhance global well-being and economic stability [75].

The post-COVID period presents a unique opportunity to rethink global mental health strategies. The pandemic highlighted the need for more flexible, innovative solutions, such as telehealth and digital mental health tools, to reach broader populations. Investment in these technologies can improve access and lower barriers to care. Additionally, allocating funds toward mental health promotion and prevention is crucial for long-term societal well-being. By increasing global mental health funding, governments and international organizations can promote a more resilient and sustainable mental health system, ensuring that mental health becomes an integral part of global health policies and recovery efforts. In our clinical case, in order to support Petros and his family, a primary care-oriented system with adequate funding and strong support for frontline practitioners is necessary.

The need for new organizational cultures that prioritize compassionate care

The COVID-19 pandemic underscored the importance of compassionate care in building resilient health systems. As healthcare workers faced immense stress, burnout, and emotional exhaustion, prioritizing compassionate care within healthcare organizations became critical to ensuring long-term resilience [81]. Compassionate care focuses on empathy, respect, and emotional support for both patients and healthcare workers, improving patient outcomes and staff well-being.

Studies show that organizations with a compassionate care culture experience higher patient satisfaction and better clinical outcomes. For example, research highlights that compassionate leadership and work environments improve job satisfaction, reduce burnout, and increase employee retention [82]. Compassionate care can also enhance patient recovery, with evidence indicating that patients who feel cared for emotionally show quicker recovery rates and better adherence to treatment [83].

In the post-COVID era, healthcare systems must integrate compassionate care into organizational structures by offering training for empathy, establishing support systems for staff, and promoting work–life balance. As healthcare systems face ongoing challenges, embedding compassionate care can improve both the quality of care provided and the mental well-being of the workforce, fostering more resilient, sustainable healthcare environments. Resembling the aftermath of the recent global economic recession, the post-COVID era suggests that compassion could once again guide healthcare systems toward a renewed direction, where reassessing professional values and services is essential to foster a more patient-centred approach [81]. This also underscores the importance of integrating compassionate care into medical education. For example, patients like Petros of our clinical scenario need an empathetic and compassionate PCP to help them navigate their suffering and anxiety.

New models for integrating mental health into primary care

The post-COVID era presents an opportunity to redefine how mental health is integrated into primary care. The pandemic has highlighted the need for accessible, flexible, and comprehensive mental health services, especially as demand for care has surged. New models for integrating mental health into primary care are essential to address this demand and improve overall health outcomes.

One promising model is the *collaborative care* approach, where mental health professionals work alongside primary care teams. Studies show that collaborative care improves patient outcomes, reduces stigma, and enhances access to mental health services. A systematic review found that this model leads to better management of depression and anxiety, with patients showing significant improvement in both mental and physical health [84].

Telemedicine has also proven effective in integrating mental health care into primary settings. Virtual consultations allow for greater accessibility, especially in rural or underserved areas. Research during the pandemic showed that telehealth services were instrumental in maintaining mental health support, with patients reporting high satisfaction, and improved access [85, 86].

Additionally, integrating digital mental health tools, such as mobile apps and online therapy platforms, can complement traditional primary care services, providing patients with self-management options. These innovative approaches ensure that mental health care is more accessible, timely, and embedded within routine healthcare, enhancing overall system resilience. In 2021, members of the WONCA Working Party on Mental Health joined World Mental Health Day in a collaborative report entitled 'Mental Health in an Unequal World: Together We Can Make a Difference', which was then produced by the World Federation for Mental Health [87]. The report endorsed several statements for shared actions on global mental health including the following:

- Primary care is exceptionally well placed to enhance mental health within universal health coverage systems.
- Family doctors are well placed to assess patients' vulnerability, the impact of poverty and disadvantage, and their association with mental and psychological conditions.
- We can intervene to reduce the mortality and morbidity of people with severe mental illness, who die prematurely often after spiraling into homelessness, unemployment, and poverty.

- We agree with the need for mental health promotion, requiring multi-sectoral collaboration to build a healthy environment with the focus on those factors that reduce chronic stress, poverty, and health inequalities.

In the clinical case of this chapter, assessing the extent to which Petros requires consultation with a psychologist or another medical specialist is crucial. Collaborative care models, successfully implemented in the United States and selected European settings, warrant increased attention. PCPs need support to address the unmet needs emerging during the post-COVID period. The digital tools that are readily available could facilitate Petros' case.

The role of telehealth and digital mental health platforms

Telehealth and digital mental health platforms have become essential tools for expanding access to mental health services, especially in the wake of the COVID-19 pandemic. These technologies offer flexible, accessible care options for patients, addressing the rising demand for mental health services while overcoming geographical and logistical barriers. According to a study, telehealth services increased by 350% during the pandemic, demonstrating their effectiveness in maintaining care continuity [88].

Digital mental health platforms, such as mobile apps and online therapy programs, also play a crucial role in promoting mental well-being. Research shows that such platforms are effective in reducing symptoms of anxiety and depression. For example, a study of an AI-powered mental health platform, reported a 14.2% reduction in depression symptoms and a 12.7% reduction in anxiety symptoms in users over a four-week period [89].

Telehealth and digital platforms also improve access for underserved populations, including those in rural areas, where mental health professionals may be scarce. A review found that telehealth interventions for depression and anxiety led to significant improvements in patient outcomes, with satisfaction rates exceeding 80%. As digital solutions evolve, they offer scalable, cost-effective models that can be integrated into traditional healthcare systems [86].

Strengthening the mental health workforce

Strengthening the mental health workforce is crucial to addressing the global mental health crisis, particularly in low- and middle-income countries where mental health professionals are scarce [68]. To address this gap, it is essential to build capacity and improve training for frontline healthcare practitioners, including PCPs, nurses, and community health workers.

A key approach is integrating mental health training into general healthcare education. Studies show that training PCPs in basic mental health care can significantly improve outcomes for patients with common mental disorders. For example, the WHO's mhGAP has demonstrated success in training primary healthcare workers in low-resource settings to manage mental health conditions, leading to improved diagnosis and treatment [67, 73]. This model has been successfully implemented in countries such as India and Uganda.

Moreover, online training platforms and digital tools can help reach a broader audience of healthcare providers. Research indicates that digital mental health training programs are cost-effective and can enhance knowledge, skills, and confidence in treating mental health issues [90–91]. By investing in workforce capacity and training, countries can ensure more sustainable, accessible mental health care globally. An opinion endorsed by the EC Expert Panel on Effective Ways of Health Investment who reported eight recommendations with several action points, among which are [7]:

- Changing of focus to mental well-being
- Treating mental well-being as an inherent part of the workplace and its organization
- Creating a supportive environment at the EU level

Public health interventions to address the global mental health challenge

Designing and evaluating public health interventions to address mental health involves campaigns aimed at reducing stigma, raising awareness, and implementing training programs to promote mental well-being. Public health campaigns, in the United Kingdom, have proven effective in reducing mental health stigma. The campaign led to a 6.6% reduction in discrimination against people with mental health issues over five years [92]. These campaigns use media, education, and community engagement to change public perceptions and encourage individuals to seek help without fear of discrimination.

Additionally, training programs focused on mental well-being and resilience are crucial for preventive care. Programs like the Mental Health First Aid in Australia provide individuals with skills to recognize early signs of mental health issues, support peers, and reduce crisis escalation. An assessment of this program showed that participants had increased confidence in handling mental health issues and better mental health literacy [93].

The evaluation of these interventions is, of course, essential to measure their effectiveness and inform future strategies. Key metrics include changes in public attitudes, mental health outcomes, and utilization of mental health services. A well-designed, evidence-based approach helps to promote long-term mental well-being and resilience across populations.

CONCLUSION

In conclusion, addressing the global mental health crisis presents significant challenges that have been magnified in the post-COVID era. The pandemic has exacerbated pre-existing mental health issues, resulting in increased rates of anxiety, depression, and suffering affecting both individuals and families. At the same time, a critical shortage of mental health professionals and inadequate funding for services remains.

To address these challenges, urgent collaboration across governments, international organizations, and the private sector is necessary. Partnerships that integrate mental health into primary healthcare systems, along with cross-border research and resource sharing, are essential to improve access and outcomes. Moreover, substantial investment in mental health infrastructure, follow-on training programs since undergraduate education, and digital solutions like telehealth and mobile apps can expand access to care, particularly in underserved regions.

Innovative strategies that focus on prevention, early intervention, and resilience-building are crucial for long-term success. By prioritizing mental health as part of the global health agenda, investing in workforce capacity, and embracing new technologies, we can create a more inclusive and resilient mental health system. Only through these concerted efforts can we effectively address the mental health challenges of today and build a healthier future for all.

REFERENCES

1. Koplan JP, Bond TC, Merson MH, Reddy KS, Rodriguez MH, Sewankambo NK, et al. Towards a common definition of global health. Lancet. 2009 Jun 6;373(9679): 1993–1995. doi: 10.1016/S0140-6736(09)60332-9.
2. Castelpietra G, Knudsen AKS, Agardh EE, Armocida B, Beghi M, Iburg KM, et al. The burden of mental disorders, substance use disorders and self-harm among young people in Europe, 1990–2019: findings from the Global Burden of Disease Study 2019. Lancet Reg Health Eur. 2022 Apr 1;16:100341. doi: 10.1016/j.lanepe.2022.100341.
3. Troup J, Fuhr DC, Woodward A, Sondorp E, Roberts B. Barriers and facilitators for scaling up mental health and psychosocial support interventions in low- and middle-income countries for populations affected by humanitarian crises: a systematic review. Int J Ment Health Syst. 2021 Jan 7;15(1):5. doi: 10.1186/s13033-020-00431-1.
4. Rathod S, Pinninti N, Irfan M, Gorczynski P, Rathod P, Gega L, Naeem F. Mental health service provision in low- and middle-income countries. Health Serv Insights. 2017 Mar 28;10:1178632917694350. doi: 10.1177/1178632917694350.
5. COVID-19 Mental Disorders Collaborators. Global prevalence and burden of depressive and anxiety disorders in 204 countries and territories in 2020 due to the COVID-19 pandemic. Lancet. 2021 Nov 6;398(10312):1700–1712. doi: 10.1016/S0140-6736(21)02143-7.
6. Winter R, Lavis A. The impact of COVID-19 on young People's mental health in the UK: key insights from social media using online ethnography. Int J Environ Res Public Health. 2021 Dec 30;19(1):352. doi: 10.3390/ijerph19010352.

7. European Commission. Supporting mental health of health workforce and other essential workers. Opinion of the Expert Panel on effective ways of investing in Health (EXPH). Publications Office of the European Union. Luxemburg. 2021.

8. OECD/European Union. Health at a Glance: Europe 2022: State of health in the EU cycle. OECD Publishing. Paris. 2022.

9. Epstein R. Attending: medicine, mindfulness and humanity. Scribner Edition. New York. 2017.

10. Nearchou F, Douglas E. Traumatic distress of COVID-19 and depression in the general population: exploring the role of resilience, anxiety, and hope. Int J Environ Res Public Health. 2021 Aug 11;18(16):8485. doi: 10.3390/ijerph18168485.

11. Munipalli B, Al-Soleiti M, Morris A, Rummans T. COVID-19: ramifications of the pandemic on mental health and substance abuse. Front Public Health. 2024 Jul 31; 12:1401734. doi: 10.3389/fpubh.2024.1401734. Erratum in: Front Public Health. 2024 Sep 16;12:1477635. doi: 10.3389/fpubh.2024.1477635.

12. The impact of COVID-19 on mental, neurological and substance use services: results of a rapid assessment. World Health Organization. Geneva. 2020. Licence: CC BY-NC-SA 3.0 IGO.

13. Tham WW, Sojli E, Bryant R, McAleer M. Common mental disorders and economic uncertainty: evidence from the COVID-19 pandemic in the U.S. PLoS One. 2021 Dec 2; 16(12):e0260726. doi: 10.1371/journal.pone.0260726.

14. Richter EP, Brähler E, Zenger M, Stöbel-Richter Y, Emmerich F, Junghans J, et al. Compounded effects of multiple global crises on mental health: a longitudinal study of East German adults. J Clin Med. 2024 Aug 13;13(16):4754. doi: 10.3390/jcm13164754.

15. Moitra M, Owens S, Hailemariam M, Wilson KS, Mensa-Kwao A, Gonese G, et al. Global mental health: where we are and where we are going. Curr Psychiatry Rep. 2023 Jul;25(7):301–311. doi: 10.1007/s11920-023-01426-8. Epub 2023 May 31. Erratum in: Curr Psychiatry Rep. 2023 Jul;25(7):313. doi: 10.1007/s11920-023-01434-8.

16. DiJulio B, Hamel L, Muñana C, Brodie M. Loneliness and social isolation in the United States, the United Kingdom and Japan: an international survey. Kaiser Family Foundation. 2018.

17. International Labour Organization. COVID-19 and the world of work. Second edition. Updated estimates and analysis. 2020

18. Vahratian A, Blumberg SJ, Terlizzi EP, Schiller JS. Symptoms of anxiety or depressive disorder and use of mental health care among adults during the COVID-19 pandemic - United States, August 2020-February 2021. MMWR Morb Mortal Wkly Rep. 2021 Apr 2; 70(13):490–494. doi: 10.15585/mmwr.mm7013e2.

19. Xiong LJ, Zhong BL, Cao XJ, Xiong HG, Huang M, Ding J, et al. Possible posttraumatic stress disorder in Chinese frontline healthcare workers who survived COVID-19 6 months after the COVID-19 outbreak: prevalence, correlates, and symptoms. Transl Psychiatry. 2021 Jul 5;11(1):374. doi: 10.1038/s41398-021-01503-7.

20. Cabarkapa S, Nadjidai SE, Murgier J, Ng CH. The psychological impact of COVID-19 and other viral epidemics on frontline healthcare workers and ways to address it: a rapid systematic review. Brain Behav Immun Health. 2020 Oct;8:100144. doi: 10.1016/j.bbih.2020.100144.

21. Pollock A, Campbell P, Cheyne J, Cowie J, Davis B, McCallum J, et al. Interventions to support the resilience and mental health of frontline health and social care professionals during and after a disease outbreak, epidemic or pandemic: a mixed methods systematic review. Cochrane Database Syst Rev. 2020 Nov 5;11(11):CD013779. doi: 10.1002/14651858.CD013779.

22. Serrano-Ripoll MJ, Meneses-Echavez JF, Ricci-Cabello I, Fraile-Navarro D, Fiol-deRoque MA, Pastor-Moreno G, et al. Impact of viral epidemic outbreaks on mental

health of healthcare workers: a rapid systematic review and meta-analysis. J Affect Disord. 2020 Dec 1;277:347–357. doi: 10.1016/j.jad.2020.08.034.

23. Collins C, Clays E, Van Poel E, Cholewa J, Tripkovic K, Nessler K, et al. Distress and wellbeing among general practitioners in 33 countries during COVID-19: results from the cross-sectional PRICOV-19 study to inform health system interventions. Int J Environ Res Public Health. 2022 May 6;19(9):5675. doi: 10.3390/ijerph19095675.

24. Soler JK, Yaman H, Esteva M, Dobbs F, Asenova RS, Katic M, et al. Burnout in European family doctors: the EGPRN study. Fam Pract. 2008 Aug;25(4):245–265. doi: 10.1093/fampra/cmn038.

25. Batra K, Singh TP, Sharma M, Batra R, Schvaneveldt N. Investigating the psychological impact of COVID-19 among healthcare workers: a meta-analysis. Int J Environ Res Public Health. 2020 Dec 5;17(23):9096. doi: 10.3390/ijerph17239096.

26. Werdecker L, Esch T. Burnout, satisfaction and happiness among German general practitioners (GPs): a cross-sectional survey on health resources and stressors. PLoS One. 2021 Jun 18;16(6):e0253447. doi: 10.1371/journal.pone.0253447.

27. Etheridge B, Spantig L. The gender gap in mental well-being at the onset of the COVID-19 pandemic: evidence from the UK. Eur Econ Rev. 2022 Jun;145:104114. doi: 10.1016/j.euroecorev.2022.104114.

28. Scheel-Hincke LL, Ahrenfeldt LJ, Andersen-Ranberg K. Sex differences in activity and health changes following COVID-19 in Europe-results from the SHARE COVID-19 survey. Eur J Public Health. 2021 Dec 1;31(6):1281–1284. doi: 10.1093/eurpub/ckab096.

29. Wester CT, Bovil T, Scheel-Hincke LL, Ahrenfeldt LJ, Möller S, Andersen-Ranberg K. Longitudinal changes in mental health following the COVID-19 lockdown: results from the survey of health, ageing, and retirement in Europe. Ann Epidemiol. 2022 Oct;74:21–30. doi: 10.1016/j.annepidem.2022.05.010.

30. Pérès K, Ouvrard C, Koleck M, Rascle N, Dartigues JF, Bergua V, Amieva H. Living in rural area: a protective factor for A negative experience of the lockdown and the COVID-19 crisis in the oldest old population? Int J Geriatr Psychiatry. 2021 Dec;36(12):1950–1958. doi: 10.1002/gps.5609.

31. Rodríguez M, Camacho JA. Rural-urban differences in the perceived impact of COVID-19 on mental health by European women. Arch Womens Ment Health. 2024 Aug;27(4):547–555. doi: 10.1007/s00737-024-01443-3.

32. Almeida M, Shrestha AD, Stojanac D, Miller LJ. The impact of the COVID-19 pandemic on women's mental health. Arch Womens Ment Health. 2020 Dec;23(6):741–748. doi: 10.1007/s00737-020-01092-2.

33. Sevilla A, Smith S. Baby steps: the gender division of childcare during the COVID-19 pandemic. Oxf Rev Econ Policy. 2020;36(Supplement_1):S169–S186.

34. Edwards KM. Intimate partner violence and the rural-urban-suburban divide: myth or reality? A critical review of the literature. Trauma Violence Abuse. 2015 Jul;16(3):359–373. doi: 10.1177/1524838014557289.

35. Racine N, McArthur BA, Cooke JE, Eirich R, Zhu J, Madigan S. Global prevalence of depressive and anxiety symptoms in children and adolescents during COVID-19: a meta-analysis. JAMA Pediatr. 2021 Nov 1;175(11):1142–1150. doi: 10.1001/jamapediatrics.2021.2482.

36. World Health Organization. COVID-19 pandemic triggers 25% increase in prevalence of anxiety and depression worldwide. 2022. Available from: https://www.who.int/news/item/02-03-2022-covid-19-pandemic-triggers-25-increase-in-prevalence-of-anxiety-and-depression-worldwide

37. UNICEF Data Hub. COVID-19 and children. Available from: https://data.unicef.org/covid-19-and-children/

38. Prommas P, Lwin KS, Chen YC, Hyakutake M, Ghaznavi C, Sakamoto H, et al. The impact of social isolation from COVID-19-related public health measures on cognitive

function and mental health among older adults: a systematic review and meta-analysis. Ageing Res Rev. 2023 Mar;85:101839. doi: 10.1016/j.arr.2022.101839.

39. Sepúlveda-Loyola W, Rodríguez-Sánchez I, Pérez-Rodríguez P, Ganz F, Torralba R, Oliveira DV, Rodríguez-Mañas L. Impact of social isolation due to COVID-19 on health in older people: mental and physical effects and recommendations. J Nutr Health Aging. 2020;24(9):938–947. doi: 10.1007/s12603-020-1469-2.

40. van Tilburg TG, Steinmetz S, Stolte E, van der Roest H, de Vries DH. Loneliness and mental health during the COVID-19 pandemic: a study among Dutch older adults. J Gerontol B Psychol Sci Soc Sci. 2021 Aug 13;76(7):e249–e255. doi: 10.1093/geronb/gbaa111.

41. Dziedzic B, Idzik A, Kobos E, Sienkiewicz Z, Kryczka T, Fidecki W, Wysokiński M. Loneliness and mental health among the elderly in Poland during the COVID-19 pandemic. BMC Public Health. 2021 Nov 2;21(1):1976. doi: 10.1186/s12889-021-12029-4.

42. Zhand N, Joober R. Implications of the COVID-19 pandemic for patients with schizophrenia spectrum disorders: narrative review. BJPsych Open. 2021 Jan 12;7(1):e35. doi: 10.1192/bjo.2020.157.

43. Ettman CK, Abdalla SM, Cohen GH, Sampson L, Vivier PM, Galea S. Prevalence of depression symptoms in US adults before and during the COVID-19 pandemic. JAMA Netw Open. 2020 Sep 1;3(9):e2019686. doi: 10.1001/jamanetworkopen.2020.19686.

44. Hastie CE, Lowe DJ, McAuley A, Mills NL, Winter AJ, Black C, et al. True prevalence of long-COVID in a nationwide, population cohort study. Nat Commun. 2023 Nov 30;14(1):7892. doi: 10.1038/s41467-023-43661-w.

45. Movahed E, Afsharmanesh A, Aqarabi H, Raesi R, Hushmandi K, Daneshi S. Comparison of the trend of suicide before and after the COVID-19 pandemic in Southeast Iran from 2016 to 2023. BMC Public Health. 2025 Jan 7;25(1):66. doi: 10.1186/s12889-024-21265-3.

46. Min S, Jeong YH, Kim J, Koo JW, Ahn YM. The aftermath: post-pandemic psychiatric implications of the COVID-19 pandemic, a South Korean perspective. Front Psychiatry. 2021 Oct 21;12:671722. doi: 10.3389/fpsyt.2021.671722.

47. Manchia M, Gathier AW, Yapici-Eser H, Schmidt MV, de Quervain D, van Amelsvoort T, et al. The impact of the prolonged COVID-19 pandemic on stress resilience and mental health: a critical review across waves. Eur Neuropsychopharmacol. 2022 Feb;55:22–83. doi: 10.1016/j.euroneuro.2021.10.864. Epub 2021 Oct 29.

48. Zhu Y, Li Y, Xu X. Suicidal ideation and suicide attempts in psychiatric patients during the COVID-19: a systematic review and meta-analysis. Psychiatry Res. 2022 Nov;317:114837. doi: 10.1016/j.psychres.2022.114837.

49. Yan Y, Hou J, Li Q, Yu NX. Suicide before and during the COVID-19 pandemic: a systematic review with meta-analysis. Int J Environ Res Public Health. 2023 Feb 14;20(4):3346. doi: 10.3390/ijerph20043346.

50. UN Women. The Shadow Pandemic: Violence against women during COVID-19. 2021. Available from: https://www.unwomen.org/en/news/in-focus/in-focus-gender-equality-in-covid-19-response/violence-against-women-during-covid-19

51. European Commission. Health at a Glance: Europe 2022. 2022. Available from: https://health.ec.europa.eu/state-health-eu/health-glance-europe/health-glance-europe-2022_en

52. McGrath JJ, Al-Hamzawi A, Alonso J, Altwaijri Y, Andrade LH, Bromet EJ, et al. Age of onset and cumulative risk of mental disorders: a cross-national analysis of population surveys from 29 countries. Lancet Psychiatry. 2023 Sep;10(9):668–681. doi: 10.1016/S2215-0366(23)00193-1.

53. Twenge J, Blanchflower D. Declining life satisfaction and happiness among young adults in six English-speaking countries. National Bureau of Economic Research. 2025,

54. World Health Organization. 2021. Available from: thttps://www.who.int/news/item/08-10-2021-who-report-highlights-global-shortfall-in-investment-in-mental-health

55. Henking C, Reeves A, Chrisinger B. Global inequalities in mental health problems: understanding the predictors of lifetime prevalence, treatment utilisation and perceived helpfulness across 111 countries. Prev Med. 2023 Dec;177:107769. doi: 10.1016/j.ypmed.2023.107769.

56. OECD. A new benchmark for Mental Health Systems. Tackling the social and economic costs of mental ill-health. OECD Health Policy Studies. OECD Publishing. Paris. 2021.

57. OECD. The unequal impact of COVID-19: A spotlight on frontline workers, migrants and racial/ethnic minorities. OECD Policy Responses to Coronavirus (COVID-19). OECD Publishing. Paris. 2022.

58. Gemelas J, Davison J, Keltner C, Ing S. Inequities in employment by race, ethnicity, and sector during COVID-19. J Racial Ethn Health Disparities. 2022 Feb;9(1):350–355. doi: 10.1007/s40615-021-00963-3.

59. Haro-Ramos AY, Brown TT, Deardorff J, Aguilera A, Pollack Porter KM, Rodriguez HP. Frontline work and racial disparities in social and economic pandemic stressors during the first COVID-19 surge. Health Serv Res. 2023 Aug;58 Suppl 2(Suppl 2): 186–197. doi: 10.1111/1475-6773.14136.

60. Camara C, Surkan PJ, Van Der Waerden J, Tortelli A, Downes N, Vuillermoz C, Melchior M. COVID-19-related mental health difficulties among marginalised populations: a literature review. Glob Ment Health (Camb). 2022 Dec 9;10:e2. doi: 10.1017/gmh.2022.56.

61. Brooks JM, Patton C, Maroukel S, Perez AM, Levanda L. The differential impact of COVID-19 on mental health: implications of ethnicity, sexual orientation, and disability status in the United States. Front Psychol. 2022 Sep 13;13:902094. doi: 10.3389/fpsyg.2022.902094.

62. Shechter A, Norful AA. A peripandemic examination of health care worker burnout and implications for clinical practice, education, and research. JAMA Netw Open. 2022 Sep 1;5(9):e2232757. doi: 10.1001/jamanetworkopen.2022.32757.

63. Koutsouri AK, Gkentzi D, Paraskevas T, Michailides C, Papantoniou K, Kavvousanos M, et al. Burnout among healthcare workers during COVID-19 pandemic: results from seven hospitals in Western Greece. Mater Sociomed. 2023;35(4):285–289. doi: 10.5455/msm.2023.35.285-289.

64. Kirzinger A, Kearney A, Hamel L, Brodie M. KFF/The Washington post frontline health care workers. Kaiser Family Foundation. 2021.

65. World Health Organization. Mental Health Atlas 2017. Geneva. 2018. Licence: CC BY-NC-SA 3.0 IGO.

66. Patel V, Saxena S, Lund C, Thornicroft G, Baingana F, Bolton P, et al. The Lancet Commission on global mental health and sustainable development. Lancet. 2018 Oct 27;392(10157):1553–1598. doi: 10.1016/S0140-6736(18)31612-X.

67. Mental Health Gap Action Programme (mhGAP) guideline for mental, neurological and substance use disorders. World Health Organization. Geneva. 2023. Licence: CC BY-NC-SA 3.0 IGO.

68. Mental Health Atlas 2020. World Health Organization. Geneva. 2021. Licence: CC BY-NC-SA 3.0 IGO

69. World Health Organization. Mental health and COVID-19. 2022. Available from: https://www.who.int/teams/mental-health-and-substance-use/mental-health-and-covid-19

70. Ran MS, Hall BJ, Su TT, Prawira B, Breth-Petersen M, Li XH, Zhang TM. Stigma of mental illness and cultural factors in Pacific Rim region: a systematic review. BMC Psychiatry. 2021 Jan 7;21(1):8. doi: 10.1186/s12888-020-02991-5.

71. Zhou W, Yu Y, Yang M, Chen L, Xiao S. Policy development and challenges of global mental health: a systematic review of published studies of national-level mental health policies. BMC Psychiatry. 2018 May 18;18(1):138. doi: 10.1186/s12888-018-1711-1.

72. World Health Organization. The Mental Health Coalition: a WHO/Europe flagship initiative. Available from: https://www.who.int/europe/publications/the-mental-health-coalition–a-who-europe-flagship-initiative?utm_source=chatgpt.com

73. World Health Organization. Mental Health Gap Action Programme (mhGAP). 2018. 2023. Available from: https://www.who.int/teams/mental-health-and-substance-use/treatment-care/mental-health-gap-action-programme

74. Fitzpatrick KK, Darcy A, Vierhile M. Delivering cognitive behavior therapy to young adults with symptoms of depression and anxiety using a fully automated conversational agent (Woebot): a randomized controlled trial. JMIR Ment Health. 2017 Jun 6;4(2):e19. doi: 10.2196/mental.7785.

75. NHS England. The five year forward view for mental health. 2016.

76. OECD. The COVID-19 pandemic and the future of telemedicine. OECD health policy studies. OECD Publishing. Paris. 2023.

77. World Health Organization. Mental health: Strengthening our response. 2018. Available from: https://www.who.int/news-room/fact-sheets/detail/mental-health-strengthening-our-response

78. World Health Organization. Mental Health Action Plan 2013–2020. Geneva. 2013.

79. Chisholm D, Sweeny K, Sheehan P, Rasmussen B, Smit F, Cuijpers P, Saxena S. Scaling-up treatment of depression and anxiety: a global return on investment analysis. Lancet Psychiatry. 2016 May;3(5):415–424. doi: 10.1016/S2215-0366(16)30024-4.

80. Lionis C. Why and how is compassion necessary to provide good healthcare? Comments from an academic physician comment on "why and how is compassion necessary to provide good quality healthcare?" Int J Health Policy Manag. 2015 Jul 15;4(11):771–772. doi: 10.15171/ijhpm.2015.132.

81. de Zulueta PC. Developing compassionate leadership in health care: an integrative review. J Healthc Leadersh. 2015 Dec 18;8:1–10. doi: 10.2147/JHL.S93724.

82. Tehranineshat B, Rakhshan M, Torabizadeh C, Fararouei M. Compassionate care in healthcare systems: a systematic review. J Natl Med Assoc. 2019 Oct;111(5):546–554. doi: 10.1016/j.jnma.2019.04.002.

83. World Health Organization and WONCA. Integrating mental health into primary care. A global perspective. 2008.

84. Bower P, Gilbody S, Richards D, Fletcher J, Sutton A. Collaborative care for depression in primary care. Making sense of a complex intervention: systematic review and meta-regression. Br J Psychiatry. 2006 Dec;189:484–493. doi: 10.1192/bjp.bp.106.023655.

85. Philippe TJ, Sikder N, Jackson A, Koblanski ME, Liow E, Pilarinos A, Vasarhelyi K. Digital health interventions for delivery of mental health care: systematic and comprehensive meta-review. JMIR Ment Health. 2022 May 12;9(5):e35159. doi: 10.2196/35159.

86. Babbage CM, Jackson GM, Davies EB, Nixon E. Self-help digital interventions targeted at improving psychological well-being in young people with perceived or clinically diagnosed reduced well-being: systematic review. JMIR Ment Health. 2022 Aug 26;9(8):e25716. doi: 10.2196/25716.

87. World Federation for Mental Health. Mental health in an unequal world: together we can make a difference. 2021.

88. Kim J, Aryee LMD, Bang H, Prajogo S, Choi YK, Hoch JS, Prado EL. Effectiveness of digital mental health tools to reduce depressive and anxiety symptoms in low- and middle-income countries: systematic review and meta-analysis. JMIR Ment Health. 2023 Mar 20;10:e43066. doi: 10.2196/43066.

89. Gega L, Jankovic D, Saramago P, Marshall D, Dawson S, Brabyn S, et al. Digital interventions in mental health: evidence syntheses and economic modelling. Health Technol Assess. 2022 Jan;26(1):1–182. doi: 10.3310/RCTI6942.

90. Mudiyanselage KWW, De Santis KK, Jörg F, Saleem M, Stewart R, Zeeb H, Busse H. The effectiveness of mental health interventions involving non-specialists and digital technology in low-and middle-income countries – a systematic review. BMC Public Health. 2024 Jan 3;24(1):77. doi: 10.1186/s12889-023-17417-6.

91. Mitchell LM, Joshi U, Patel V, Lu C, Naslund JA. Economic evaluations of internet-based psychological interventions for anxiety disorders and depression: a systematic review. J Affect Disord. 2021 Apr 1;284:157–182. doi: 10.1016/j.jad.2021.01.092.

92. Evans-Lacko S, Corker E, Williams P, Henderson C, Thornicroft G. Effect of the time to change anti-stigma campaign on trends in mental-illness-related public stigma among the English population in 2003-13: an analysis of survey data. Lancet Psychiatry. 2014 Jul;1(2):121–8. doi: 10.1016/S2215-0366(14)70243-3.

93. Kitchener BA, Jorm AF. Mental health first aid training for the public: evaluation of effects on knowledge, attitudes and helping behavior. BMC Psychiatry. 2002 Oct 1;2:10. doi: 10.1186/1471-244x-2-10.

SECTION 2

CHAPTER 4

Mental health and remote consultations

Transferring evidence and experience to low-resource settings

Flávio Dias Silva, Darien Alfa Cipta, and Ferdinando Petrazzuoli

INTRODUCTION

A woman visits a family doctor seeking help for her brother, Cameron. Since the end of school time, he, a 29-year-old man, has had a small electronic devices repair store, and usually spends his time working, and twice a week visiting his family. He never married or had children. In the last year, after a brother's death, he started with persecutory ideas - men in black cars were supposed to be trying to kill him. In the last two months, Cameron has started to become more isolated from his family, and now he does not leave his house, worried about those men. His sister tries to take her brother to a doctor's office, but he does not want to get out of his house for fear of being murdered. She says his thoughts seem fragmented, and his hygiene has declined greatly, going several days without showering. Cameron does not feel comfortable welcoming any health worker to visit him at home. However, he agrees to see a doctor by video call.

Remote consultations in family medicine have been a helpful tool in providing broader access to patients, especially during and after the COVID-19 pandemic. Despite there being few robust studies, 'telemedicine' has been shown to improve the quality of patient care; is feasible through several methods like

DOI: 10.1201/9781003473947-7

consultation by telephone, mail, video call, or combinations of these; and has been associated with significant patient satisfaction [1]. On the other hand, virtual mental health consultations are not a very recent technology – as early as 1973 Thomas Dwyer [2] published a paper about the development of an 'interactive television (IA TV) system set up between Massachusetts General Hospital and a medical station in Boston'. He said that 'the system has proven to be feasible and acceptable to individuals and institutions in the community, providing psychiatric skills on a much wider scale, in a more accessible way, and faster than any other system' [2].

The advance and spreading access to videoconferencing by the internet has made the 'at distance' communication between doctors and patients easier and more powerful. Remote consultations have been a great instrument for a potential revolution in healthcare because they can offer a solution for places where there are few (or no) doctors or other health professionals. Especially in the mental health field, where the world suffers from a huge professional gap, and clinical practice is not so dependent on physical examination, remote consultations can be a strong tool for access to care. To put into practice this technology, of course, depends on overcoming a lot of challenges. Local regulation issues regarding ethics and data safety, technological requirements such as the internet, appropriate software, and electronic device availability, as well as adequate consultation setting, are only some aspects in planning the delivery of this service. However, all these elements can be affordable with some investment. It is noteworthy that in addition to remote consultations, the internet can offer plenty of resources for mental health care to underserved populations. The field called Digital Health also involves the possibilities of mobile app prescription and virtual and/or augmented virtuality therapeutic use and has been met with significant enthusiasm.

REMOTE CONSULTATIONS IN MENTAL HEALTH CARE

Conducting medical consultations at a distance using information technology and communication has been a reality for some decades in several countries [3], and so it has been in the field of psychiatry [4, 5]. In the mental health care field, 'telepsychiatry', i.e., at-distance psychiatric visits, is like face-to-face care in diagnostic reliability and clinical outcome measures [6, 7]: satisfactory for professionals and patients [6, 8, 9], and more cost-effective than in-person care [6, 10]. This has been true in different group populations and health settings, such as clinics, hospitals, and homes [5]. In addition to remote psychiatric care, other at-distance mental health interventions have proven to be effective, such as psychotherapy [11], synchronous and asynchronous contacts through messaging via cell phone, email exchanges, phone calls, and even support groups through virtual meetings by chat or videoconferences [12]. In a meta-analysis of 184 randomised controlled studies, online Cognitive-Behavioural Therapy (CBT) was shown to be effective, especially for problems such as depression and anxiety disorders [13]. There are also robust studies about strategies for integrating mental health care with primary care through teleconsultations among professionals [14] and even computerisation of integrated care models [15]. In Brazil, the Telehealth Brazil Network Program has developed a wide range of actions on integrating care since 2007 [16], some leading to important improvements in the availability of specialized services.

Despite all this evidence, it was only after the COVID pandemic that telemedicine began to be widely used. A study in the United States, a country that had already regulated this practice before 2020, reveals that there was an increase in the use of teleconsultations of 766% in the first three months of the pandemic, and from 0.3% of all interactions in March to June 2019 to 23.6% of all interactions in the same period in 2020 [17]. A report by the Organisation for Economic Co-operation and Development (OECD), which has 38 member countries worldwide, reports that the picture was similar in several other nations. Pre-pandemic restrictions on the use of telemedicine were relaxed at the beginning of 2020, and some countries have even used financial incentives to boost telemedicine. However, the telemedicine policies introduced with the pandemic are still temporary in most countries and lack definitive regulation [18].

All this considered, remote consultations have proven to have the potential to be a very strong resource for caring for people who have difficulty accessing a doctor's surgery. In addition, information and communication technologies can improve the quality of standard face-to-face care by increasing doctor–patient interaction. Electronic pre-consultation forms, contact between sessions via internet-based chat applications and the use of e-mail for clinical purposes are examples of resources already used by some professionals. The challenge has been to offer all these possibilities in a structured way that is adapted to the patient's needs.

Standards for evaluation of services that offer remote consultations have been proposed for some institutions like the Pan American Health Organization [19] and the American Telemedicine Association [20]. The latter, in an expert panel review, built a lexicon of 36 aspects clustered in four groups to consider how to assess a telemedicine service (Table 4.1). Paying attention to these indicators seems to be a good starting point to offer a qualified service.

A number of questionnaires have been developed and used to evaluate telemedicine from patient and provider perspectives. They can be very helpful to evaluate the implementation of a service and guide needed improvements. Most of them assess patient and provider satisfaction, and usability of systems,

TABLE 4.1 American Telemedicine Association Lexicon for Telemedicine Services Evaluation

• **Patient Satisfaction**	• No shows	• *Economic evaluation (standard models and using the below indicators):*	• Patient safety
• **Provider Satisfaction**	• Accuracy of assessment	• Value proposition	
• **Coordination of care**	• Symptom outcomes	• Travel direct costs	
• **Integration of care**	• Completion of treatment	• Travel indirect costs	
• **Usability**	• Quality of care	• Technology direct costs	
• **Rapport**	• Treatment utilization	• Technology direct costs	
• **Stigma**	• Number of services	• Public vs. private	
• **Motivational Readiness**	• Numbers served	• Cost avoidance	
	• Wait times	• Missed obligations	
	• Length of session	• Burden on social network	
	• Distance to service	• Personnel costs	
	• Likelihood to access vs. traditional care	• Supplies costs	
	• Cultural access	• Training costs	
		• Facilities and maintenance	
		• Broad resource utilization	

Source: Compiled by the authors, based on Shore et al., 2014.

sometimes in a combined way. Telehealth Usability Questionnaire (TUQ), Telemedicine Satisfaction Questionnaire (TSQ), and Service User Technology Acceptability Questionnaire (SUTAQ) have been the most specific telemedicine questionnaires used in recent research; however, other non-specific instruments evalutate users' satisfaction, usability, and acceptance of technology, as the Client Satisfaction Questionnaire (CSQ), Questionnaire for User Interaction Satisfaction (QUIS), System Usability Scale (SUS), Patient Satisfaction Questionnaire (PSQ), and Technology Acceptance Model (TAM) [21]. The TUQ [22] was designed to be a comprehensive questionnaire that covers all usability factors (i.e., usefulness, ease of use, effectiveness, reliability, and satisfaction) and assesses 21 perceptions in a 7-point Likert scale from 'Disagree' to 'Agree' (Box 4.1). It can be used to obtain patients' and doctors' perspectives.

BOX 4.1 COMPONENTS OF TELEHEALTH USABILITY QUESTIONNAIRE

- Telehealth improves my access to healthcare services.
- Telehealth saves me time travelling to a hospital or specialist clinic.
- Telehealth provides for my healthcare needs.

- It was simple to use this system.
- It was easy to learn to use the system.
- I believe I could become productive quickly using this system.
- The way I interact with this system is pleasant.
- I like using the system.
- The system is simple and easy to understand.
- This system can do everything I would want it to be able to do.
- I can easily talk to the clinician using the telehealth system.
- I can hear the clinician using the telehealth system.
- I felt I was able to express myself effectively.
- Using the telehealth system, I can see the clinician as well as if we met in person.
- I think the visits provided over the telehealth system are the same as in-person visits.
- Whenever I made a mistake using the system, I could recover easily and quickly.
- The system gave error messages that clearly told me how to fix problems.
- I feel comfortable communicating with the clinician using the telehealth system.
- Telehealth is an acceptable way to receive healthcare services.
- I would use telehealth services again.
- Overall, I am satisfied with this telehealth system.

Source: Compiled by the authors, based on Parmanto et al. [22].

ESSENTIAL ASPECTS IN DELIVERING TELE-MENTAL HEALTH CARE

Cameron's sister contacts her family physician and asks him for a remote consultation for her brother. The family doctor says that he is afraid that maybe he cannot help the patient, but they agree that at least a screening could be made by video call. The doctor starts to think about what the best standards are to make this encounter the most like a face-to-face one, and how he can establish a trusting relationship with the patient since he has never been trained to perform tele-mental health care.

Hardware, software, and internet

A good quality data transmission (audio, video) is essential for similarity to face-to-face assessments. Usually, currently, mobile phones as well as computers are equipped with cameras and headphones/microphones with enough technology to make good quality calls. These can be a feasible option for patients who need remote consultations from home. In some cases, however, patients may go to a medical or technology facility (e.g., Lan house) to establish a connection with the remote doctor; in these cases, additional hardware technology could be a stand-alone camera, a device that permits the doctor to control the patient camera and amplifies the doctor's view of the patient, allowing zoom and entire patient body perspective. On the other hand, internet can be accessed by cable, mobile internet offered by telecommunication companies, and by satellite. The latter is a potentially groundbreaking technology that can reach the most remote locations in the globe. Internet speed to make video calls can be as low as 128 kbps, but for a better quality of data transmission, at least 300 kbps is recommended. Finally, there is plenty of software to make video calls, some non-specific and others especially developed for medical consultations. The most important requirement is safety against data leaking. American authorities recommend that software used to make video calls must comply with the HIPPA (Health Insurance Portability and Accountability Act) requirements (https://www.hhs.gov/hipaa/for-professionals/index.html). These requirements may vary from country to country and are of extreme importance to prevent transmission of the consultation to people other than the doctor and the patient. Also, other ways of conducting internet-based telemedicine (e.g., mail and chats) must follow these guidelines. Additionally, all these tools could be especially robust against data leakage if they were integrated into the patient's electronic health record.

Legal issues

Remote consultations are regulated in somewhat different ways in different countries. In some places, like Indonesia, first consultations are recommended to be in person. In Brazil, although first consultations are allowed remotely, caring for chronic conditions requires at least one face-to-face visit each no more than 180 days. In the United States, phone (only audio) psychiatric consultations were recently allowed as a way of maintaining treatment, and it can be the only form of talking with the doctor for up to 12 months after an in-person visit. Electronic prescription of drugs also may vary in countries, and not all medications can be dispensed by pharmacies through this method.

International remote consultations are a special topic to be discussed. This can be a helpful resource for migrants to keep being cared for by their compatriot doctors, but it is fundamental to respect local regulations for practising medicine. Usually, doctors must be licensed to see a patient in each country, even by remote consultations. However, collaborating with local doctors in a consultation-liaison model can be an alternative to providing important transcultural support for immigrant/displaced people. Prescriptions of medicines (whether in paper or electronic format) usually are not valid in other countries, but this is changing in Europe, where at least Spain, Portugal, Estonia, Croatia, Poland, and Finland adopted international validation of electronic prescriptions (https://health.ec.europa.eu/ehealth-digital-health-and-care/electronic-cross-border-health-services_en). Given this, remote consultation services must be planned considering local regulations.

On the other hand, considering the importance of the above-mentioned issues, one of the most important legal requirements to perform telemedicine is obtaining a consent form from the patient. This is the tool that will provide official information about the remote consultation procedure, explaining the process, its characteristics and limits, its digital safety issues, and establishing a clear plan for the eventual need to escalate/refer to in-person consultation. The World Psychiatric Association Telepsychiatry Global Guidelines [23] has proposed the main components of a consent form as displayed in Box 4.2.

BOX 4.2 ELEMENTS OF A REMOTE CONSULTATION CONSENT FORM

- Legal base of remote consultations in the country
- Need to offer a phone number of a relative who can be reached in case of emergency
- Software used
- Orientation that the patient has to be in a private place without the presence of other people, except those that they want, or the professional considers necessary
- Remembering to not record consultations unless previously agreed
- Explanation of the eventual need for a personal visit to complement evaluation or to get prescriptions unavailable by electronic methods
- A backup plan, in case of internet problems

Note: All this information could be available in a short video with spoken information, in addition to the written document, which would be very helpful to a patient's understanding of the consultation characteristics.

Source: Compiled by the authors based on 'The World Psychiatric Association Telepsychiatry Global Guidelines' (Mucic, Shore & Hilty, 2024).

There is no absolute contraindication to remote consultations. However, it is important that providers take into account the appropriateness of the service for each individual patient, considering factors that may make the virtual visit difficult. According to World Psychiatric Association guidelines [23], this includes the patient's cognitive capacity, their history regarding cooperativeness with treatment professionals, their current and past difficulties with substance abuse, and their history of violence or self-injurious behaviour; in addition, providers must consider the geographic distance to the nearest emergency medical facility, the efficacy of the patient's support system, and the patient's current medical status.

Setting – virtual clinics and provider skills in teleconsultations

Remote consultations must have the same professionalism as in-person visits. Privacy must be guaranteed on both sides of the virtual meeting; it is recommended that patients and doctors be in safe and comfortable rooms. Sometimes the use of earphones can be of importance to a better sense of commitment. Image and sound standards must be cautiously prepared; the doctor must avoid excessive distractors in the background, try to have a neutral colour environment and be in the centre of the screen, with eyes at the level of the camera. Additionally, the doctor's screen can be instantaneously shared with the patient to explain test results, for example. Despite this, little data is available about the specific skills that a professional must develop to offer optimal teleconsultations. Digital literacy, adaptability to different software, flexibility to jump from virtual to in-person in the same agenda, communication skills (verbal, non-verbal, and written or multimedia), and coaching the patient through the virtual experience (e.g., helping to adjust camera focus) seem important abilities that a health professional should develop.

It should be noted that it can be more difficult to establish a therapeutic and trustful relationship remotely. Lack of provider skills accounts in part for this difficulty, but patient issues like sensory deficits (hearing, seeing), or even the burden that dealing with technology can elicit for both patient and doctor must be considered. Some tips have been suggested to create a more therapeutic alliance between doctors and patients in virtual meetings [23]:

- Asking where the patient is and trying to understand their context and culture could be a good initiative. Knowing where the patient is can also help to call local police/ambulance services for emergency intervention to save a patient's life (attempted suicide) or someone else's life (homicidal attempt).
- Personalizing greetings and using charts to augment communication (like 'yes' or 'no' charts) can bring a little humour to the interaction and bridge the gap imposed by physical distance.
- An important drawback is the relative lack of non-verbal cues between patients and doctors, maybe asking a patient to stand upright in front of the camera can be, in some cases, a way of evaluating movement and posture issues.
- Ensure the patient is in a safe, quiet, comfortable space to optimize the attention and presence of both parties. It is recommended that the patient not be in a public space, but in a private room, whenever it is available. The therapist needs to assess the 'spatiality', the space, and the overall environment the client inhabits.
- Try to anticipate the possible disruption of a poor internet connection and provide an alternative means to connect.

DIGITAL HEALTH – OTHER CONTRIBUTIONS OF THE TECHNOLOGY TO MENTAL HEALTH CARE

Cameron was assessed by the family physician. Besides understanding that the patient's persecutory ideas were delusions, and his thoughts and behaviour were moderately disorganized, the doctor noted the flat affection of the patient and his poor self-care. The physician then diagnosed a primarily psychotic disorder and prescribed risperidone. In addition, he recommended that the patient must start to practise some techniques for anxiety and sleep hygiene using a mobile application designed for behavioural therapy. Four weeks later, Cameron went to the doctor's office, less anxious and paranoid, and agreed to start broader psychosocial care in a specialized centre.

Mobile application prescriptions

Numerous applications have been developed for helping in the management of mental problems. This includes mental disorder digital screening and monitoring tools, and therapeutic electronic resources, delivered as unsupervised use programmes, professional/peer-oriented programmes, and even as electronic games. Digital health is indeed a field of service delivery with a huge potential to help to diminish the mental health professional gap worldwide.

On the other hand, the efficacy of a few programmes contrasts with a lack of evidence of several new start-ups and applications providing elements of mental health care, which is fuelled by a growing commercial interest. The first skill that doctors must develop to prescribe these resources is to know what already proven applications exist, their limitations due to language and cultural differences, and how to evaluate the evidence base of each one. In addition, some have drawn attention to the potential worsening of the burden of care with new technologies, to both doctors and patients [24]. It seems important that investigations be made about to what extent digital transformation can lead to 'digital stress', especially for those patients with less technological skills or who suffer from multimorbidity/polypharmacy, and, on the other hand, for doctors with already burdensome practices. Finally, important international institutions are worried about the ethical risks of disruptive technology on mental health regarding, for example, exacerbation of behavioural traits such as social withdrawal and isolation, and more severely, disclosure of personal health information online, where it may be accessed by relatives, friends, employers or others, and have unintended social and consequences for the patient [25].

Table 4.2 displays some evidence-based applications used in mental health care.

Virtual and/or augmented reality

Virtual reality (VR) is a cutting-edge technology capable of immersing users in a simulated environment created by computer systems. It achieves this by engaging the user's visual, auditory, and sometimes even tactile senses, providing a fully immersive experience, often using specialized headsets and stereoscopic displays. Although VR has primarily been associated with entertainment, particularly in the gaming industry, its applications have expanded to the realm of mental health care. In recent years, VR has emerged as a promising tool for remote mental health consultation in primary care settings. Therapeutic VR experiences have been developed and tested to address a wide range of mental health concerns. One area where VR has demonstrated significant potential is in the treatment of specific phobias. Numerous studies have explored the use of VR therapy to help individuals confront and overcome their fears, such as fear of flying or arachnophobia [38]. These VR experiences can be customised to create controlled, immersive scenarios that allow patients to confront their fears gradually and safely, leading to desensitization and therapeutic progress.

TABLE 4.2 Some mobile applications that have been demonstrated to help people with mental problems, and their applicability

Application	App type	Aims	Target population	Evidence of efficacy by PsyberGuide	Language/Country availability	References
Peak (Brain Training)	Cognitive training	Enhance well-being, schizophrenia & psychosis	MCI in elderly	2.86/5 (0.57)B	Worldwide	[26]
Lumosity	Cognitive training	Enhance cognitive abilities	MCI in older adults	3.21/5 (0.64)A	Worldwide	[27]
Headspace	Meditation	Enhance well-being, anxiety & manage stress, support a child's mental health	Teens to adults	4.64/5 (0.93)A	English, French, German, Spanish & Portuguese	[28]
Calm	Mindfulness, Meditation	Enhance well-being, manage anxiety & stress, support a child's mental health	Children, teens, adults, older adults	2.85/5 (0.57)B	Worldwide (English)	[29]
Relax Melodies: Sleep Sounds	Meditation	Enhance quality of sleep, meditation programmes	Children, teens, adults, older adults	–	English, Spanish	[30]
FABULOUS (Self-Care)	Behaviour tracker, health coach, emotional well-being	Create, strengthen, and track healthy habits	Teens, adults	1.43/5 (0.29)C	Paris, France	[31,32]

(Continued)

TABLE 4.2 Some mobile applications that have been demonstrated to help people with mental problems, and their applicability *(Continued)*

Application	App type	Aims	Target population	Evidence of efficacy by PsyberGuide	Language/Country availability	References
Pacifica	Meditation, mood tracking, peer support, emotional support	Enhance well-being, overcome depression, manage anxiety & stress	Teen to adult	2.85/5 (0.57)B	Worldwide (English)	[33]
Stop, Breathe, and Think	Meditation, mindfulness	Enhance well-being, manage anxiety & stress	Teens, adults, older adults	2.50/5 (0.50)B	Worldwide (English)	[34]
Insight Timer	Meditation, mindfulness	Enhance well-being, overcome depression, manage anxiety & stress	Adults, older adults	2.50/5 (0.50)B	Worldwide	[35]
Daylio	Tracker (mood journal)	Enhance well-being, overcome depression, & manage anxiety & stress	Teen, adults, older adults	2.10/5 (0.42)C	Worldwide	[36, 37]

Source: Compiled by authors.

App ratings in this table were sourced from PsyberGuide, a nonprofit project of One Mind that provides expert reviews of mental health applications based on credibility, user experience, and data transparency. The platform remains publicly accessible and has been referenced in peer-reviewed literature (e.g., Garland et al., *Family Systems & Health*, 2021;39(1):155–157). However, readers should note that the frequency of updates to app evaluations may vary.

Augmented reality (AR), on the other hand, integrates virtual content seamlessly into real-world environments using cameras and display devices. It overlays virtual elements onto the physical surroundings, effectively blending the boundaries between the digital and real worlds. Notably, the mobile game 'Pokémon Go' showcased the potential of AR technology by encouraging users to explore their physical surroundings while hunting for digital creatures. In the field of mental health care, AR presents exciting possibilities for enhancing remote consultations in primary care. By utilizing AR applications and wearable devices, primary care physicians and mental health professionals can offer real-time support and guidance to patients in their own environments. For instance, patients can receive augmented reality-based guidance for managing anxiety or practising mindfulness exercises in their daily lives. The interactive and personalized nature of AR interventions can facilitate engagement and adherence to treatment plans, ultimately contributing to better mental health outcomes. As the boundaries of VR and AR technology continue to expand, the integration of these immersive technologies into primary care settings holds the potential to revolutionise the delivery of mental health care, making it more accessible, engaging, and effective for patients. On the opposite side, it is important to highlight that a recent meta-analysis showed that 62% of studies on VR/AR did not address the adverse effects of these technologies [39]. These findings indicate that future studies must monitor the worsening of mental health outcomes (like psychosis or worsening social anxiety) and the eventual emergence of other health problems – like the case with the increase in crash injuries related to Pokémon GO a few years ago [40].

The integration of AR and VR technology into primary care, particularly in low- to middle-income countries, presents a range of formidable barriers [41]. Access to high-quality VR and AR hardware may be limited in resource-constrained settings, hindering widespread adoption. The substantial costs associated with equipment, software, and maintenance pose financial challenges for healthcare facilities and patients alike. Ensuring healthcare providers possess the requisite skills and training to effectively utilize AR and VR is vital for successful implementation. Patient engagement with and acceptance of these technologies varies, making it crucial to address comfort and willingness to use AR and VR as part of mental health treatment. Protecting patient data privacy within virtual environments is paramount, necessitating robust security measures. Navigating regulatory and ethical considerations, which often lag technology advancements, is a central challenge. In socio-culturally diverse low- to middle-income countries, language and cultural differences can introduce unique complexities in design and delivery [42]. Ensuring cultural sensitivity and accessibility to individuals from diverse backgrounds is essential. Pragmatic trials are instrumental in addressing these challenges and assessing the real-world effectiveness of AR and VR in primary care, offering insights into the practicality, feasibility, patient outcomes, and cost-effectiveness of these technologies. Such trials inform policymakers, healthcare providers, and researchers, enabling the development of effective strategies for harnessing AR and VR in mental health care, ultimately improving access and the quality of care, even in low- to middle-income countries.

RECOMMENDATIONS

Telemedicine has advantages compared to in-person consultations in providing care where there is a lack of or non-available mental health care (psychiatry and/or clinical psychologist). In remote areas, there is often a lack of specialist doctors, making telemedicine valuable. On the other hand, challenges include low patient and family awareness, high consultation costs, and medication delivery issues. In addition, telemedicine is primarily used by newcomers or non-indigenous people. Although telehealth has the potential to bridge a gap, rural areas may have limited internet access or technological literacy. The absence of broadband internet and lack of computer technology compatible with telehealth hampers the uptake of telehealth in many rural communities [43, 44]. Moreover, it cannot fully replace face-to-face care [45].

Considering all the recent experience accumulated in telemedicine and tele-mental health care, some essential recommendations appear to be very helpful in establishing a remote consultation service:

- Offer video call consultations as a resource, as well as opportunities for digital literacy learning for staff and communities, especially among rural populations.
- Consider the availability of a structured office for remote consultations in the local health facility, what can be of value to provide the consultation with general doctors (where there is no one), or with secondary care, in a liaison model, including with transcultural specialists.
- Before the consultation, obtain written consent, and know where the patients are from, and where local resources are in case of emergency referral.
- Consider establishing a pre- and post-consultation service through one of the following technologies: mail, chat, or telephone. Pre-consultation could offer history-taking data collection by electronic forms linked to electronic health records. Post-consultation could be a reasonable option for receiving complementary tests requested by the doctor in the consultation, as well as for orientations about test results and patient follow-up.

- Evaluate periodically the service using validated questionnaires, but also qualitative data, being aware of patients' and professionals' perspectives. Assess clinical and quality outcomes.
- Incorporate prescription of digital tools – mobile apps, VR, and AR devices – only after careful evidence assessment and monitoring of positive and negative effects.

FURTHER READING AND e-RESOURCES

- e-Mental Health. Davor Mucic, Donald M. Hilty. https://doi.org/10.1007/978-3-319-20852-7. Springer Cham. 2015, 310p
- Digital Mental Health: A Practitioner's Guide. Ives Cavalcante Passos, Francisco Diego Rabelo-da-Ponte, Flavio Kapczinski. https://doi.org/10.1007/978-3-031-10698-9. Springer Cham. 2023. 259p
- American Psychiatry Association Telepsychiatry toolkit. Available on https://www.psychiatry.org/psychiatrists/practice/telepsychiatry
- DIGA (Digital Health App Directory), a governmental German guide to select evidence-based apps. https://diga.bfarm.de/de

REFERENCES

1. Vodička S, Zelko E. Remote consultations in general practice-a systematic review. Zdr Varst. 2022;61. https://doi.org/10.2478/sjph-2022-0030
2. Dwyer TF. Telepsychiatry: psychiatric consultation by interactive television. Am J Psychiatry. 1973;130. https://doi.org/10.1176/ajp.130.8.865
3 Harzheim E, Fernandes JG. Guia_Avaliacao_telessaude_telemedicina. 2017;82.
4. Bashshur RL, Shannon GW, Bashshur N, et al. The empirical evidence for telemedicine interventions in mental disorders. Telemed J e-Health. 2016;22:87–113.
5. Hilty DM, Ferrer DC, Parish MB, et al. The effectiveness of telemental health: a 2013 review. Telemed J e-Health. 2013;19:444–454.
6. Hubley S, Lynch SB, Schneck C, et al. Review of key telepsychiatry outcomes. World J Psychiatry. 2016;6:269.
7. De Las Cuevas C, Arredondo MT, Cabrera MF, et al. Randomized clinical trial of telepsychiatry through videoconference versus face-to-face conventional psychiatric treatment. Telemed J e-Health. 2006;12:341–350.
8. Kruse CS, Krowski N, Rodriguez B, et al. Telehealth and patient satisfaction: a systematic review and narrative analysis. BMJ Open. 2017;7:1–12.
9. Nguyen M, Waller M, Pandya A, et al. A review of patient and provider satisfaction with telemedicine. Curr Allergy Asthma Rep. 2020;20. https://doi.org/10.1007/s11882-020-00969-7
10. Grady BJ A comparative cost analysis of an integrated military telemental health-care service. Telemed J E Health. 2002;8:293–300.
11. Simon PD. A quick review of recommendations and evidences on telepsychotherapy and digital psychiatry for researchers and mental health professionals in the time of COVID-19. Int J Soc Psychiatry. 2021 Aug;67(5):604–605. https://doi.org/10.1177/0020764020962537
12. Langarizadeh M, Tabatabaei MS, Tavakol K, et al. Telemental health care, an effective alternative to conventional mental care: a systematic review. Acta Inform Med. 2017;25:240–246.
13. Zainal NH, Soh CP, Van Doren N, Benjet C. Do the effects of internet-delivered cognitive-behavioral therapy (i-CBT) last after a year and beyond? A meta-analysis of

154 randomized controlled trials (RCTs). Clin Psychol Rev. 2024 Nov 16;114:102518. https://doi.org/10.1016/j.cpr.2024.102518

14. Liddy C, Drosinis P, Keely E. Electronic consultation systems: worldwide prevalence and their impact on patient care-a systematic review. Fam Pract. 2016;33:274–285.

15. Fortney JC, Pyne JM, Mouden SB, et al. Practice-based versus telemedicine-based collaborative care for depression in rural federally qualified health centers: a pragmatic randomized comparative effectiveness trial. Am J Psychiatry. 2016;170:414–425.

16. Shaver J. The state of telehealth before and after the COVID-19 pandemic. Prim Care. 2022 Dec;49(4):517–530. https://doi.org/10.1016/j.pop.2022.04.002

17. OECD. "The future of telemedicine after COVID-19", OECD Policy Responses to Coronavirus (COVID-19), OECD Publishing, Paris. 2023. https://doi.org/10.1787/d46e9a02-en

18. Schmitz CAA, Harzheim E. Oferta e utilização de teleconsultorias para Atenção Primária à Saúde no Programa Telessaúde Brasil Redes. Rev Bras Med Fam Comunidade. 2017;12:1–11.

19. PAHO. Defining evaluation indicators for telemedicine as a tool for reducing health inequities. 2016.

20. Shore JH, Mishkind MC, Bernard J, et al. A lexicon of assessment and outcome measures for telemental health. Telemed e-Health. 2014;20:282–292.

21. Hajesmaeel-Gohari S, Bahaadinbeigy K. The most used questionnaires for evaluating telemedicine services. BMC Med Inform Decis Mak. 2021;21:1–11.

22. Parmanto B, Lewis AN Jr, Graham KM, et al. Development of the Telehealth Usability Questionnaire (TUQ). Int J Telerehabil. 2016;8. https://doi.org/10.5195/ijt.2016.6196

23. Mucic, D, Shore, J, Hilty, D. The World Psychiatric Association Telepsychiatry Global Guidelines. J Technol Behav Sci. 2024;9:572–579. https://doi.org/10.1007/s41347-023-00339-w

24. Mair FS, Montori VM, May CR. Digital transformation could increase the burden of treatment on patients. The BMJ. 2021;375. https://doi.org/10.1136/bmj.n2909

25. World Economic Forum. Global Governance Toolkit for Digital Mental Health: Building Trust in Disruptive Technology for Mental Health April 2021. 2021. https://www3.weforum.org/docs/WEF_Global_Governance_Toolkit_for_Digital_Mental_Health_2021.pdf (accessed 15 December 2023)

26. Bonnechère B, Klass M, Langley C, et al. Brain training using cognitive apps can improve cognitive performance and processing speed in older adults. Sci Rep. 2021;11. https://doi.org/10.1038/s41598-021-91867-z

27. Ballesteros S, Mayas J, Prieto A, et al. A randomized controlled trial of brain training with non-action video games in older adults: results of the 3-month follow-up. Front Aging Neurosci. 2015;7. https://doi.org/10.3389/fnagi.2015.00045

28. Champion L, Economides M, Chandler C. The efficacy of A brief app-based mindfulness intervention on psychosocial outcomes in healthy adults: a pilot randomised controlled trial. PLoS One. 2018;13. https://doi.org/10.1371/journal.pone.0209482

29. Huberty J, Green J, Glissmann C, et al. Efficacy of the mindfulness meditation mobile app "calm" to reduce stress among college students: randomized controlled trial. JMIR Mhealth Uhealth. 2019;7. https://doi.org/10.2196/14273

30. Weekly T, Walker N, Beck J, Akers S, Weaver M. A review of apps for calming, relaxation, and mindfulness interventions for pediatric palliative care patients. Children (Basel). 2018 Jan 26;5(2):16. https://doi.org/10.3390/children5020016

31. Cantisano LM, Gonzalez-Soltero R, Blanco-Fernández A, Belando-Pedreño N. ePSICONUT: An e-health programme to improve emotional health and lifestyle in university students. Int J Environ Res Public Health. 2022 Jul 28;19(15):9253. https://doi.org/10.3390/ijerph19159253

32. Carlo AD, Hosseini Ghomi R, Renn BN, et al. Assessment of real-world use of behavioral health mobile applications by a novel stickiness metric. JAMA Netw Open. 2020;3. https://doi.org/10.1001/jamanetworkopen.2020.11978

33. Moberg C, Niles A, Beermann D. Guided self-help works: randomized waitlist controlled trial of Pacifica, a mobile app integrating cognitive behavioral therapy and mindfulness for stress, anxiety, and depression. J Med Internet Res. 2019;21. https://doi.org/10.2196/12556

34. Athanas AJ, McCorrison JM, Smalley S, et al. Association between improvement in baseline mood and long-term use of a mindfulness and meditation app: observational study. JMIR Ment Health. 2019;6. https://doi.org/10.2196/12617

35. O'Donnell KT, Dunbar M, Speelman DL. Effectiveness of using A meditation app in reducing anxiety and improving well-being during the COVID-19 pandemic: a structured summary of A study protocol for A randomized controlled trial. Trials. 2020;21. https://doi.org/10.1186/s13063-020-04935-6

36. Chaudhry BM. Daylio: mood-quantification for a less stressful you. Mhealth. 2016;2. https://doi.org/10.21037/mhealth.2016.08.04

37. Cristol S. Patient's perspective on using mobile technology as an aid to psychotherapy. JMIR Ment Health. 2018;5. https://doi.org/10.2196/10015

38. Gottlieb A, Doniger GM, Hussein Y, et al. The efficacy of a virtual reality exposure therapy treatment for fear of flying: a retrospective study. Front Psychol. 2021;12. https://doi.org/10.3389/fpsyg.2021.641393

39. Lundin RM, Yeap Y, Menkes DB. Adverse effects of virtual and augmented reality interventions in psychiatry: systematic review. JMIR Ment Health. 2023;10. https://doi.org/10.2196/43240

40. Richards KG, Wong KY, Khan M. Augmented reality game-related injury. BMJ Case Rep. 2018;11. https://doi.org/10.1136/bcr-2017-224012

41. Kouijzer MMTE, Kip H, Bouman YHA, et al. Implementation of virtual reality in healthcare: a scoping review on the implementation process of virtual reality in various healthcare settings. Implement Sci Commun. 2023;4. https://doi.org/10.1186/s43058-023-00442-2

42. Pimentel D, Foxman M, Davis DZ, et al. virtually real, but not quite there: social and economic barriers to meeting virtual reality's true potential for mental health. Front Virtual Real. 2021;2. https://doi.org/10.3389/frvir.2021.627059

43. Graves JM, Abshire DA, Koontz E, Mackelprang JL. Identifying challenges and solutions for improving access to mental health services for rural youth: insights from adult community members. Int J Environ Res Public Health. 2024;21(6):725.

44. Graves JM, Mackelprang JL, Amiri S, Abshire DA. Barriers to telemedicine implementation in Southwest tribal communities during COVID-19. J Rural Health. 2021;37(1):239.

45. Perkins D, Farmer J, Salvador-Carulla L, Dalton H, Luscombe G. The orange declaration on rural and remote mental health. Aust J Rural Health. 2019;27(5):374–379.

CHAPTER 5

Mental health for primary care professionals

The role and leadership of management and health systems in mental health promotion in working settings

Darien Alfa Cipta, Natasya Reina, Dyta Ghezhanny William, Juan Mendive, Heather L. Rogers, and Ferdinando Petrazzuoli

CASE STORY – BURNOUT IN A FAMILY DOCTOR

Dr. Maria P., a 52-year-old primary care physician, had been practising for 25 years in a busy urban clinic. She is married and has two children. Known for her dedication, empathy, and thoroughness, she was beloved by her patients and colleagues alike. Over the years, however, increasing administrative burdens, electronic medical record (EMR) requirements, and a growing patient load began to weigh heavily on her.

Maria started feeling perpetually drained, even after weekends or vacations. The thought of returning to work filled her with dread.

She noticed herself becoming detached from her patients. Instead of feeling compassion, she often felt numb or irritated.

DOI: 10.1201/9781003473947-8

Despite working long hours, Maria felt like she was barely making a difference. The endless paperwork seemed more significant than patient care, leaving her feeling ineffective and disillusioned.

One afternoon, Maria made a minor error in prescribing medication. Although the issue was quickly corrected, she was consumed by guilt and anxiety. That evening, she broke down at home, admitting to her spouse that she felt trapped and unable to continue.

Encouraged by her family and a trusted colleague, Maria sought support.

She began seeing a psychologist specializing in healthcare worker burnout, who helped her recognize the symptoms and underlying causes. Maria worked with a coach to establish boundaries and develop time-management skills tailored to her high-pressure environment. Joining a peer support group for physicians helped Maria share her experiences and gain perspective.

Maria's clinic also played a role in her recovery. The clinic hired additional administrative staff to handle documentation and EMR-related tasks. Maria transitioned to a four-day workweek. The clinic introduced mindfulness programs and scheduled regular check-ins to monitor staff well-being.

After several months, Maria felt a renewed sense of purpose. While she acknowledged the challenges of primary care, she now had the tools to cope. Her relationships with her patients improved, and she found joy in medicine again.

Dr. Maria's case highlights the importance of recognizing burnout early, seeking help, and addressing both personal and systemic factors. Burnout is not a personal failure, but a signal that change is needed for both the individual and the healthcare system.

INTRODUCTION

Concern about mental health in the workplace has been rising in recent years, and, especially as a result of the pandemic, among healthcare workers specifically. Levels of burnout, moral injury, and mental disorders, including suicide among physicians, are notably high, and can no longer be ignored by healthcare leadership. This chapter seeks to explain the factors contributing to the mental health and well-being of primary care physicians (PCPs) in their workplaces. The importance of interventions at multiple levels, including individual factors, job characteristics, organizational aspects, and societal context will be examined. Case studies to illustrate the benefits of interventions at different levels will be presented. Furthermore, this chapter introduces a metric not commonly used to measure organizational performance – the compassion aspect of the institution – as an essential indicator of a safe working environment. Leadership and teamwork with multidisciplinary professionals play a key role in institutionalizing compassion in daily clinical practice and running the business of healthcare organizations.

DEFINING MENTAL WELL-BEING FOR PCPs AND RELATED FACTORS

The subject of mental health and well-being has emerged as one of the most frequently discussed topics among various academic and non-academic resources. Each workplace has its own risk and related factors that may lead to declining mental health. Undeniably, the healthcare system is also affected by this problem. It has been found that 20% to 50% of internationally studied physicians reported experiencing burnout, characterized by depersonalization and emotional exhaustion [1]. Another study revealed that even before COVID-19, 32% to 80% of doctors were at a high risk of 'burnout' [2]. According to the World Health Organization (WHO), burnout is defined as a syndrome resulting from chronic workplace stress that has not been successfully managed. Burnout may lead to feelings of energy depletion, increased mental distance or negativism, and reduced professional efficacy [3].

Burnout is also an important concern regarding patient safety. The healthcare sector is one of the fields that necessitates minimal potential errors in its professional practice. Undesirable circumstances, such as medical errors, unwarranted medical care orders, and early leave from the medical profession are more likely to happen among physicians experiencing burnout. Unfortunately, up to this day, there is no agreed definition of mental well-being universally among clinicians.

A 2018 systematic review sought to define physicians' well-being and a standardized measure of it [1]. This review highlighted the need for an operational definition to allow comparable measurement across different intellectual and geographical areas. Although the operational definition internationally has yet to be agreed upon and established, this study concluded that the definition of well-being was a state of positive feelings and meeting full potential in the world. Specifically, physician well-being is a multifaceted construct that includes psychological, physical, social, and emotional wellness, and spiritual health in both personal and work lives. Moreover, the literature revealed that physician wellness includes the presence of positive well-being, such as thriving states and behaviours beyond satisfaction and the absence of distress or mental disorder/illness. Figure 5.1 provides a conceptualization of a few things that might contribute to a person's well-being [3].

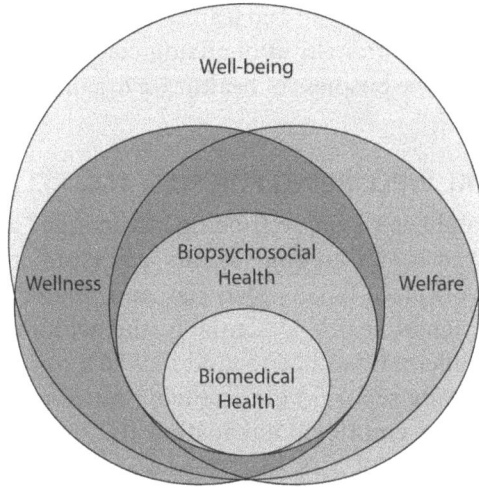

FIGURE 5.1 Concept diagram of mental well-being [2].

Healthcare is a complex, highly regulated, and demanding field that requires full attention of all healthcare practitioners, with PCPs being the first line of defence. Therefore, it is important for PCPs to have a strong emotional resilience or stable emotional state as one of the fundamental aspects of mental well-being to handle work-related stressors. Resilience refers to the ability to cope with stressors and challenges in the medical field, such as facing patients with diverse medical conditions, delivering bad news, and managing uncertainty. Developing emotional resilience is crucial to ensure PCPs can provide compassionate care without being overwhelmed. Other than that, psychological health is equally important, where PCPs find fulfilment in their profession and view their work as meaningful. Furthermore, social support contributes to psychological health and resilience, in that PCPS need to have someone to lean on and someone who understands the challenges of their workload. A study in Turkey showed that positive emotions, good quality of sleep, and life satisfaction were associated with increased psychological resilience of 214 healthcare workers during the COVID-19 pandemic [4]. Prioritizing the mental well-being of PCPs is not only essential for personal health, but it acts as a cornerstone of quality patient care where it is closely linked to their capacity to provide compassionate and competent care.

RISK AND PROTECTIVE FACTORS OF BURNOUT, MORAL INJURY, AND MENTAL DISORDERS AMONG PCPs

In order to support the mental well-being of PCPs, risk factors that might be a potential threat must be identified. Heavy workloads (high volume of patients, long or irregular shifts, high pace, insufficient resources, extensive administrative tasks), lack of psychological or physical safety, workplace-related bullying, moral conflicts, perceived job security, and lack of social support are a few factors that can contribute to the elevated stress among healthcare workers. Other than that, limited resources, government, corporate micromanagement, negative media reports, and threats of law involvement regarding errors can also be big threats for PCPs. It is critical to investigate and act on this work-related stress to maintain the well-being of healthcare workers. Burnout is also associated with work-to-family conflicts, personal issues, unrealistic expectations of patients, ongoing pressure of lifelong learning and updating knowledge, and poor communication among healthcare professionals [5]. The WHO estimates a shortfall of 18 million health workers, primarily in low- and lower middle-income countries by 2030. Also, the ratio of overall population and healthcare workers in low and lower middle-income countries is another major issue which adds to healthcare workers' work burden, stress, and burnout [5, 6].

Ethical dilemmas and moral injury are additional related issues that healthcare workers may face while providing care. Moral injury is defined as psychological distress that results from actions, or the absence of action, that violate someone's moral or ethical code. This might cause a feeling of guilt when someone's decisions or actions do not align with one's own moral values and beliefs. The situation where a healthcare worker has to make important and difficult decisions, such as choosing who will get to be put on a ventilator, end-of-life care decisions, or withholding certain treatments are a few examples of situations that might lead to moral injury. People who have developed moral damage are likely to see themselves negatively and question their own actions. This may lead to negative thoughts and significant negative health impacts, including leaving the healthcare profession and in some cases, leading to suicidal ideation [5].

Moral injury can potentially lead to mental illness, such as depression, post-traumatic stress, anxiety, insomnia, and even suicidal ideation. The overall rate of suicide attempts among physicians is 1%, with 17% reporting suicidal thoughts [5]. This worsened during the COVID-19 pandemic, especially in low- and middle-income countries (LMICs) where PCPs were struggling to meet the overwhelming demands while their own physical safety was not guaranteed. A global review of the COVID-19 pandemic showed a high incidence of anxiety disorders at 23% and depression at around 27% among primary healthcare frontliners. In total, about 70% of medical healthcare suffered from anxiety, whereas 50% experienced depression. Another systematic review stated that the pooled prevalence of depression for frontline professionals was approximately 25% [5].

These findings underscore the importance of the government or corporate leadership to make changes that effectively address the mental well-being of PCPs. PCPs are at risk of experiencing burnout, moral injury, and mental disorders due to the demanding nature of their profession. People have to occasionally be reminded that PCPs are also human beings whose resilience has limits and are also vulnerable as human beings.

MULTI-LEVEL INTERVENTIONS FOR IMPROVING WELL-BEING

With the identification of issues at hand, it is vital to begin the search for a solution. Enhancing mental well-being in the healthcare sector can be achieved through a holistic approach or multi-level interventions which consist of individual, organizational, and community initiatives. These interventions are rooted in the understanding that individual well-being is profoundly influenced by the surrounding environment. Interventions can be divided into two groups: those that focus on internal self-improvement and those that modify external environmental factors.

Internal self-improvement can be achieved by practising self-care which involves self-compassion, self-awareness, self-altruism, and implementing it across physical, social, and inner self-care domains [5]. Frequently, prioritizing self-care is not a common practice among clinicians, as they are trained to put the patient first. It is undeniable that some clinicians may fear being judged or feel selfish when they think about taking care of their own needs. Recent reviews state that self-care is the first line of defence for healthcare workers, especially in balancing one's personal needs and the needs of others [7]. Maintaining a healthy lifestyle that includes regular exercise, adequate sleep, recreational activities and hobbies, and practising mindfulness and meditation are a few of the most effective self-care strategies. It is also important to be more selective of the relationships around the individual PCP. Healthy and close relationships, such as those with family, should be prioritized. Physicians are encouraged to focus on their strengths, instead of engaging in self-critical thinking about things that could have been done better. To avoid accumulation of stress and burnout, physicians should try to prioritize and simplify tasks, seek support, and continuously monitor personal limits, as well as communicate assertively. The beneficial effects of appropriate self-care have been recorded, such as improved physical, mental, and emotional well-being, including empathy, optimism, and self-efficacy, which are vital for psychological resilience.

External environmental factors play a pivotal role in the preservation of well-being and, for workers, this can be divided into two distinct categories:

organizational and community influences. Organizational interventions involve promoting work–life balance, creating a supportive work environment, and making mental health resources and self-care tools available. During times of crisis, healthcare workers should be provided with psychological first aid and long-term support through mental health support programmes. This facilitates getting early intervention and treatment for mental disorders with confidential counselling and peer support. In response to the COVID-19 pandemic, an ideal tool that can be used to address elevated psychological stress and risk of burnout is the WHO's Self-Help Plus (SH+) stress management intervention. As an alternative, a telemedicine platform might also be a safe place where PCPs can share their opinions and experiences with one another. Managing a positive work environment is also one of the most effective ways to prevent burnout or other mental health issues among PCPs. A supportive work environment is one that attracts and encourages people to remain in the health workforce, as well as enabling effective performance and better adaptation [8]. A positive work environment is closely related to how healthcare leaders organize and promote a supportive and collaborative team, instead of one based on comparison and competition. Work–life balance is also an integral part of PCPs' mental health. Scheduling of work shifts and limiting the length of work shifts should be combined with adequate opportunities to participate in mental health support programmes. Furthermore, leave policies (e.g., parental, sick, personal development) should be in place such that they do not add additional burden to other healthcare provider's schedules.

The next category of intervention to support the well-being of PCPs involves community efforts which promote and sustain good mental health. Community well-being is a proactive force that can significantly improve mental health. It might be engaged through recreational facilities, events, and volunteer activities that might foster a sense of belonging, purpose, and fulfilment. Community health refers to a convergence of healthcare services, economics, and social responsibilities. It is an overall state of emotional, social, and physical health within a community or society [9]. PCPs should be able to choose the group of social community with whom they want to engage further. A community that reduces stigma and addresses mental health will create an environment where PCPs feel more comfortable and safer in seeking help when needed. Participating in community life, such as cultural activities or volunteering has been linked to increased mental well-being [10]. Meeting new people and connecting with others who share similar values might enhance a community identity and a sense of meaning. By allocating additional time, PCPs may experience a temporary diversion that could potentially positively affect their mental well-being and health.

In conclusion, implementing interventions at each of the levels described previously provides a holistic and comprehensive approach to enhancing the overall well-being of PCPs. Multi-level interventions consist of individual, organizational, and community programmes designed to create a positive and supportive environment that empowers PCPs to help themselves when necessary and hopefully can lead to sustainable improvement in well-being. Mental well-being is affected by various internal and external factors. Therefore, a comprehensive strategy is needed, with a focus on external supportive environments (to not blame the individuals and overmedicalize the problem too, in some instances), to fully address these influences on PCP well-being.

CASE STUDIES OF POLICY INTERVENTION (INCLUDING SOME EXAMPLES FROM THE PANDEMIC CONTEXT)

CASE STUDY 5.1 – The Ohio State Medical Center

The Ohio State health system places a strong emphasis on clinician well-being, with a focus on providing trauma recovery support and encouraging open communication among clinicians to address the social and emotional challenges they encounter while delivering care. Within the Stress, Trauma, and Resilience (STAR) Program, two key initiatives support clinician well-being: Brief Emotional Support Teams (BESTs) and Schwartz Rounds®. BESTs offer mental and emotional support to clinicians following stressful or traumatic events, facilitating debriefs and identifying individuals in need of additional support. BESTs are trained to provide immediate emotional support to clinicians and staff after stressful or traumatic events, nurturing a culture of peer support and helping to identify those in need of additional support after such events [11].

Opportunities for trauma debriefings are identified through an in-house operating line, the STAR line, which facilitates the deployment of trained trauma debriefing facilitators within 24 hours. Staff training to become BEST facilitators involves a half-day session, maintaining consistency and quality. Components of trauma debriefing include psychological first aid, crisis intervention, motivational interviewing, and cognitive reframing to help clinicians reframe harmful narratives following traumatic events. STAR Program staff follow up individually with clinicians to connect them with additional support services if needed.

Schwartz Rounds® at Ohio State is held on the first Friday of every month. These meetings are open to all clinicians and medical centre staff and typically include an average of 180 people, providing regular opportunities to discuss the social and emotional challenges they face while caring for patients and their families. These interdisciplinary sessions encourage open conversations and provide support, fostering a culture of well-being. These rounds illustrate that many clinicians share similar challenges and that they are not alone in facing them. Informal feedback surveys help shape future meetings and encourage open communication among clinicians.

The Gabbe Health and Wellness Initiative coordinates various programmes to enhance the well-being of faculty and staff. It offers a free mindfulness course, culinary medicine classes, and staff retreats. Oversight is provided by a steering committee and funding is sourced from an internal risk management grant. To gauge clinician well-being, the Ohio State health system administers a biannual engagement survey, with 'pulse surveys' conducted in off years for units with lower engagement scores. These assessments enable the health system to continually improve and prioritize clinician well-being [11].

CASE STUDY 5.2 – Singapore Ministry of Health Policies

Research in Singapore has identified significant public stigma towards those with mental illness, and people have admitted that they would not seek help for a mental health condition due to the associated stigma. To support healthcare workers in public healthcare institutions (PHIs), the Ministry of Health in Singapore has introduced measures aimed at encouraging them to seek support. They also reiterate their commitment to bolstering the mental well-being of healthcare professionals.

Healthcare staff in Singapore's healthcare clusters now have access to a comprehensive suite of services to support their mental well-being. To foster a culture of openness regarding mental health, awareness campaigns and initiatives have been initiated. These endeavours are designed to encourage healthcare staff to proactively seek assistance when necessary. Additionally, regular surveys are conducted to gauge staff morale, resilience, and their ability to cope with the various challenges they face. A pivotal facet of this initiative is the introduction of new training programmes focused on mental wellness. These programmes are mandatory for all public healthcare staff, ensuring that they possess the requisite knowledge and tools to effectively manage their mental well-being. Furthermore, making attendance at the training obligatory helps to reduce the stigma with seeking out these types of programmes and services.

Leveraging technological advancements, PHIs have implemented online self-assessment tools and artificial intelligence (AI) chatbots, such as Wysa and BotMD. These innovative solutions facilitate early intervention, preventing the deterioration of mental well-being among healthcare workers. These channels empower healthcare staff to raise concerns regarding the mental well-being and safety of their colleagues or they themselves, with a commitment to prompt issue resolution.

The support network for healthcare professionals has been further expanded through the strengthening of peer-support networks. This expansion now includes department well-being champions, fostering open discussions and a sense of community. This initiative offers a much-needed listening ear and support for those in need. The Ministry of Health continues to collaborate with PHIs to advocate for mental health awareness and support mental wellness initiatives. The overarching goal is to foster a culture that encourages healthcare staff to consistently seek the support they need to safeguard their mental well-being within a supportive structure that enhances resilience.

THE ROLE OF LEADERSHIP IN INSTITUTIONALIZING COMPASSION IN PRIMARY CARE ORGANIZATIONS
Compassion in primary care organizations

In the complex world of healthcare, the importance of compassion in fostering a culture of well-being and excellence cannot be overstated. Compassion in primary care organizations extends beyond the individual acts of kindness by healthcare providers; it represents a systemic commitment embedded within organizational culture, leadership, and policies. Compassionate care encompasses psychological, emotional, social, and spiritual well-being for both patients and healthcare providers, ensuring that care delivery is humanistic, sustainable, and equitable [12].

The role of leadership in institutionalizing compassion

Leadership is pivotal in embedding compassion into the core fabric of primary care organizations. Beyond driving organizational success and meeting performance targets, leaders have a profound influence on the professional satisfaction and mental health of the physicians they oversee. Research demonstrates that effective leadership behaviours can significantly reduce burnout and enhance job satisfaction among healthcare professionals. For instance, a 2013 study conducted at the Mayo Clinic found that every 1-point increase in leadership score (on a 60-point scale) correlated with a 3.5% decrease in burnout likelihood and a 9.1% increase in job satisfaction [12].

To institutionalize compassion, leaders must actively support their teams through:

- *Recognizing Individual Talents*: Physicians who dedicate at least 20% of their time to meaningful work are at a significantly lower risk of burnout. Leaders should identify and facilitate opportunities for such engagement.
- *Regular Leadership Assessments*: Leadership evaluations should include feedback on how leaders promote well-being and compassion, alongside traditional performance metrics.
- *Strategic Leadership Changes*: Leaders who fail to meet compassionate leadership standards despite mentorship may need to be replaced to ensure organizational integrity, and faithful to the vision and mission of the body [13, 14].

Compassionate compensation models

Traditional productivity-based compensation models often clash with the principles of compassionate care. These models can incentivize overwork, leading to burnout, and diminished care quality. Organizations should consider alternative models that prioritize physician well-being, such as:

- *Salaried Compensation*: Offering fixed salaries to mitigate the pressure of productivity targets.
- *Multi-Dimensional Metrics*: Incorporating patient satisfaction, quality measures, and meaningful work time into compensation criteria.
- *Flexibility and Support*: Facilitating work–life balance through flexible scheduling and protected time for personal growth, mentorship, and community engagement [13, 14].

Training and education for compassion

Educational initiatives are crucial for fostering a culture of compassion. Training programmes should begin early in medical education and extend throughout a physician's career. Innovative approaches, such as narrative medicine, mindfulness practices, and interdisciplinary workshops, can enhance relational and interpersonal skills. Moreover, compassion training should not be limited to clinical staff, but should also include administrative and managerial teams to create an organization-wide ethos of care [13, 14].

Sustaining a compassionate organizational culture

Institutional compassion requires ongoing commitment and strategic planning. Regular assessments of organizational culture, refresher courses for healthcare teams, and platforms for emotional reflection (e.g., Schwartz Rounds®) are essential. Compassion must also be integrated into performance evaluations and institutional benchmarks to maintain its relevance amidst competing priorities. Leaders must ensure that policies support not only patient care, but also the holistic well-being of their teams.

Compassionate care is not merely an idealistic goal, but a practical strategy for improving healthcare outcomes, reducing burnout, and fostering professional fulfilment. By prioritizing compassion in leadership, education, and organizational policies, primary care organizations can create a sustainable, supportive, and effective healthcare system [13, 14].

BALINT GROUPS AS A THERAPEUTIC OASIS

The term Balint groups is derived from the name of the psychoanalyst Michael Balint (1896–1970). During the late 1950s, Michael Balint and his wife Enid initiated psychological training workshops for general practitioners (GPs) in London. Their approach was documented in the book titled *The Doctor, His Patient and the Illness* published in 1957. In these workshops, traditional lectures were replaced with a format centred on the presentation and discussion of medical cases in small groups of around nine to ten participants, led by a psychoanalyst [15].

Participation in Balint groups is consistently reported as a cost-effective and easily implementable approach, even without extensive organizational support. These groups, as supported by numerous studies, contribute to the improvement of communication skills and foster participants' awareness of their psychological processes. Furthermore, they have a positive impact on doctors' perceptions of their patients' issues, enhancing their interpersonal skills and deepening their understanding of their emotional well-being. The gatherings typically last 60–90 minutes and involve six to ten individuals led by a coordinator. During a session, one participant presents a case with personal and emotional significance, along with associated questions and issues. While the presenter steps back from the discussion, the other members engage in empathetic discussions, avoiding direct advice, criticism, or reproach. The presenting individual re-enters the group at the end to provide feedback [16].

Balint groups aim to enhance the emotional competence, empathy, and relational skills of healthcare professionals and prevent stress-related disorders. They have been shown to significantly improve physicians' emotional competence, self-awareness, and job satisfaction. These groups also foster a sense of professional and human solidarity among members, reducing feelings of isolation and loneliness. Importantly, Balint groups are considered an effective and practical method for preventing burnout and its progression. The formation of this circular group, where doctors gathered to discuss shared concerns in an empathetic and supportive environment, brought a significant change to their work dynamics. Typically isolated in their rooms behind desks and computers, seeing patients one after another, doctors worked within a rigid professional and administrative hierarchy. In contrast, the group had no hierarchy, and the leaders aimed to guide rather than instruct.

In Balint activity, the group itself may be seen as an area for adult play, a playground in which the leaders create a safe and consistent system for experimentation and interdisciplinary cooperation. By leaders encouraging 'playing' in groups, the members can feel free to be able to make appropriate choices and express mistakes. The space for playing therefore serves as a therapeutic function, a place for potential experimenting and exploring new innovations and possibilities within the clinician–patient relationship, as well as the member–group–leader interface. Playfulness in Balint encounters may also encourage intimacy and group cohesion. This 'group space' should be open, non-threatening, and supportive, enabling the presenter and the group to reflect and develop, through play and experimentation, questioning often rigid internal structures.

A study in Romania aimed to measure the potential impact of Balint groups in physicians [17]. The study's findings indicated that individuals who participated in Balint groups exhibited a reduced tendency to utilize denial and self-blame as coping mechanisms. Instead, they showed a greater inclination to seek emotional and practical support. Additionally, these participants reported higher scores in terms of experiencing pleasurable emotions with low arousal, positive emotions, and perceiving a sense of meaning in their lives. However, when accounting for other factors such as gender and age, the unique impact of Balint training appeared to primarily influence the preference for specific coping strategies. These results may encourage the incorporation of Balint groups into physician training programmes.

CONCLUSION

In a traditional medical culture where hard work and sacrifice values are often emphasized in professionalism, evidence supports positive outcomes when healthcare leaders pay attention to workplace mental health issues. Balancing the dialectics of dedication-to-patient and self-care as an integral part of professionalism, reinforced by institutionalized compassion in the organization, is key. Although further research and analysis in this area is warranted, best practices as outlined in this chapter are promising avenues for replication, transfer to new workplaces, and scaling up.

KEY POINTS

- Physician well-being can be defined as a state of positive feelings and meeting full potential in the world that includes psychological, physical, social, and emotional wellness, and spiritual health in both personal and work lives.
- Factors associated with physician mental health include burnout, moral injury, and symptoms of mental disorders, such as anxiety, depression, suicidal ideation, and post-traumatic stress disorder. Psychological resilience is an important protective factor.
- Effective interventions to improve physician mental health and well-being are often multi-level, aiming to modify associated individual-level, organizational-level, and community-level factors.
- Stress management interventions are examples of individual-level interventions to enhance physician well-being.
- Organizational changes that can improve physician well-being include scheduling modifications, controlling patient demand, offering managerial and/or peer support, and reducing the stigma surrounding coming forward with symptoms of distress.
- Community-level interventions aim to foster a sense of belonging, purpose, and fulfilment via, for instance, volunteering and participation in community-run activities.
- Institutional compassion is an indicator that should be included in performance metrics for healthcare organizations to encourage appropriate monitoring of physician mental well-being.

REFERENCES

1. Brady KJ, Trockel MT, Khan CT, Raj KS, Murphy ML, Bohman B, et al. What do we mean by physician wellness? A systematic review of its definition and measurement. Acad Psychiatry. 2017;42(1):94–108.
2. Simons G, Baldwin DS. A critical review of the definition of 'wellbeing' for doctors and their patients in a post-COVID-19 ERA. Int J Soc Psychiatry. 2021;67(8):984–991.
3. World Health Organization Widens the Definition of Burnout [Internet]. Prospect. 2019 [cited 2023 Oct 30]. Available from: https://prospect.org.uk/news/world-health-organisation-widens-definition-of-burnout
4. Bozdag F, Ergün N. Psychological resilience of healthcare professionals ˇ during COVID-19 pandemic. Psychol Rep. 2020:33294120965477. doi: 10.1177/0033294120965477
5. Izdebski Z, Kozakiewicz A, Białorudzki M, Dec-Pietrowska J, Mazur J. Occupational burnout in healthcare workers, stress and other symptoms of work overload during the COVID-19 pandemic in Poland. Int J Environ Res Public Health. 2023;20(3):2428.
6. Benson J, Sexton R, Dowrick C, Gibson C, Lionis C, Ferreira Veloso Gomes J, Bakola M, AlKhathami A, Nazeer S, Igoumenaki A, Usta J, Arroll B, van Weel-Baumgarten E, Allen C. Staying psychologically safe as a doctor during the COVID-19 pandemic. Fam Med Community Health. 2022 Jan;10(1):e001553. doi: 10.1136/fmch-2021-001553

7. Sanchez-Reilly S, Morrison LJ, Carey E, Bernacki R, O'Neill L, Kapo J, et al. Caring for oneself to care for others: physicians and their self-care. J Support Oncol. 2013;11:75–81. doi: 10.12788/j.suponc.0003

8. Wiskow C, Albreht T, de Pietro C. "How to create an attractive and supportive working environment for health professionals." Health Systems and Policy Analysis. 2010. Available from: http://www.euro.who.int/__data/assets/pdf_file/0018/124416/e94293. pdf

9. S. C. Community Health and Its Importance [Internet]. International Online Medical Council. International Online Medical Council (IOMC). 2021 [cited 2023 Nov 4]. Available from: https://www.iomcworld.org/open-access/community-health-and-its-importance-63417.html

10. Nichol B, Wilson R, Rodrigues A, Haighton C. Exploring the effects of volunteering on the social, mental, and physical health and well-being of volunteers: an umbrella review. Voluntas. 2023. doi: 10.1007/s11266-023-00573-z

11. Cappelucci K, Zindel M, Knight HC, Busis N, Alexander CM. Improving clinician well-being at the Ohio State University: a case study. NAM Action Collaborative on Clinician Well-Being and Resilience, National Academy of Medicine, Washington, DC. 2019. https://nam.edu/clinicianwellbeing/case-study/ohio-state-university

12. Shanafelt TD, Noseworthy JH. Executive leadership and physician well-being. Mayo Clinic Proceedings. 2017;92(1):129–146. doi: 10.1016/j.mayocp.2016.10.004

13. Shea S. Is it possible to develop a compassionate organization? comment on "why and how is compassion necessary to provide good quality healthcare?" Int J Health Policy Manag. 2015 Jun 23;4(11):769–770. doi: 10.15171/ijhpm.2015.119

14. Lionis C. Why and how is compassion necessary to provide good healthcare? comments from an academic physician comment on "why and how is compassion necessary to provide good quality healthcare?" Int J Health Policy Manag. 2015 Jul 15;4(11):771–772. doi: 10.15171/ijhpm.2015.132

15. Roberts M. Balint groups: a tool for personal and professional resilience. Can Fam Physician. 2012 Mar;58(3):245–247.

16. Rabin S, Maoz B, Shorer Y, Matalon A. Balint groups as 'shared care' in the area of mental health in primary medicine. Ment Health Fam Med. 2009 Sep;6(3):139–143.

17. Popa-Velea O, Mihăilescu AL, Diaconescu L, Gheorghe LR, Ciobanu AM. Meaning in life, subjective well-being, happiness and coping at physicians attending Balint groups: a cross-sectional study. Int J Environ Res Public Health. 2021;18(7):3455. doi: 10.3390/ijerph18073455

18. Rizal W. Supporting mental well-being of healthcare professionals amidst COVID-19 pandemic and preventing burnout [Internet]. Ministry of Health. 2022 [cited 2023]. Available from: https://www.moh.gov.sg/news-highlights/details/supporting-mental-well-being-of-healthcare-professionals-amidst-covid-19-pandemic-and-preventing-burn-out

CHAPTER 6

Priorities for primary mental care in low-resource settings

Implementing sustainable approaches to mental health care delivery in settings with traditionally low motivation for mental health care

Alfredo de Oliveira Neto, Adekunle Joseph Ariba, Abdullah Dukhail AlKhathami, and Ferdinando Petrazzuoli

INTRODUCTION

AP, a 23-year-old female undergraduate in her second year, had dreams of excelling in her academics to the extent that she hoped to graduate with a first-class degree. But by the end of the first year, she had to carry over two courses. She became withdrawn and began to experience a decline in her mental well-being and her effort to improve her psychological well-being marked the beginning of a troubling journey through the healthcare system.

AP first visited her university health clinic seeking help for what she and her family believed to be a physical ailment. She was diagnosed with typhoid and malaria, conditions that are prevalent in her community. But her symptoms – fatigue, sadness, and a lack of interest in previously enjoyed activities – did not abate. The attending primary care providers did not recognize the signs of her developing depression.

DOI: 10.1201/9781003473947-9

AP's mother took her to a church for prayer – a common intervention for illnesses perceived to defy orthodox medical care in her community. Unfortunately, even with this, PA's condition continued to deteriorate and, after much delay, she was taken to a neuropsychiatric hospital where she was finally diagnosed with severe depression.

This scenario aptly illustrates a significant mental health treatment gap prevalent in LMICs. The lack of integration of mental health care into primary care settings often leads to misdiagnosis and delayed treatment. If AP had received appropriate mental health care at the university clinic, her mild symptoms could have been addressed early on, and progression to severe depression might have been prevented.

AP's case is a touching reminder of the mental health treatment gap faced by many in LMICs. Prioritizing mental health within primary care provides a holistic healthcare approach that can address the most common forms of ailment in the community, be these physical or psychosocial.

EPIDEMIOLOGY OF MENTAL HEALTH CONDITIONS IN LOW-RESOURCE SETTINGS

Mental, neurological, and substance use (MNS) disorders constitute a major disease burden worldwide [1–3], but the greatest impact of the disease burden is felt among the nations that are resource-constrained [4, 5]. For instance, while the Mental Health Treatment Gap (mhGAP) is a global phenomenon, the gap is disproportionately wide in low-resource countries [6, 7]. In some wealthy countries, the overall treatment gap is up to 53%; but it is as high as 78% in some less resource-endowed countries of the same region [8]. The gap is even wider (up to 90%) in Africa, particularly in the sub-Saharan region [9, 10]. Reasons include the high prevalence of MNS in these countries, as well as the impact of widespread poverty [11, 12]. More than 80% of persons who have mental disorders live in LMICs, and the majority of such countries are found in Sub-Saharan Africa, Southeast Asia, Latin America, and Eastern Mediterranean Region. Not only serious mental illness (SMI), the prevalence of common mental disorders (CMDs) such as depression and anxiety is among the highest globally [18, 19].

Common features of such countries include low per capita income and widespread poverty, with about 50% of their citizens living below the poverty line [13, 14]. For example, Nigeria's per capita as at 2021 was US$2,085 while that of the United States of America was US$69,288. Worse still, Burundi, regarded as one of the least developed countries, had a gross domestic product

(GDP) of US$237 in the same year [11]. Importantly, the healthcare systems are characterized by a shortage of healthcare workers, including doctors, nurses, and other professionals. This is due to both inadequate production of such workers as well as their maldistribution locally, and emigration to wealthier nations where their services are highly appreciated and well remunerated [15]. The common health indices in these countries – particularly maternal and infant mortality – are badly affected [16]. But even worse is the mental disease burden.

MENTAL CARE SERVICE DELIVERY IN RESOURCE-CONSTRAINED NATIONS

Among LMICs the provision of mental health care services differs widely, depending on the level of development – particularly with regards to financial resources, workforce, and infrastructure. It is well established that the healthcare workforce in general is limited in LMICs, but the situation is much worse with mental health care personnel. Some of the countries have just one mental health care professional to 100,000 persons. Studies show that in the poorest countries as much as 90% of persons with severe mental disorders do not receive appropriate care [20].

Mental health care is not adequately funded globally, even in high-income countries, but the situation is much worse in LMICs where some countries allocate less than 1% of their health budget to mental health care, and most of such funding goes to specialized psychiatric centres in urban areas. At the community level, limited availability of health insurance coverage compels most patients and their families to pay out of pocket with the risk of catastrophic health expenditure. A recent systematic review that focused on the progress towards healthcare financing in LMICs using benefit and financing incidence analyses concluded that the healthcare financing in these countries benefits the rich more than the poor [21].

One major constraint is the healthcare workforce. Previous researchers have highlighted the extreme scarcity of professional healthcare personnel in LMICs [22]. Unfortunately, more recent predictions paint a gloomy picture of the future of the health workforce in these countries. It is projected that there will be a global shortage of 15 million health workers by 2030 and it is the resource-constrained nations that will bear the brunt of this shortage because their needs will exceed supply and demand [23]. As of 2020, low-income countries have on average 1.4/100,000 population mental health workers compared to 62.2/100,000 population in high-income countries [24]. This restricted workforce is a major impediment to optimal mental care service delivery in these countries.

Another barrier to optimal mental health care is the significantly low level of mental literacy in some of these countries [25]. Under such circumstances, the cultural norms may prevent people from acknowledging the presence of mental illness which may then be explained in terms of cultural and religious norms [26, 27]. The high level of stigma reported to be commonly associated with psychological disorders in such communities constitutes an additional barrier to seeking and receiving effective treatment [12]. Mental care delivery is also limited by under-representation of mental health service delivery infrastructure and capacity such as absent or obsolete referral system, up-to-date treatment guidelines, lack of integration into the overall health system, as well as poor research capacity [28].

EFFORTS TO REDUCE THE TREATMENT GAP IN MENTAL HEALTH CARE SERVICES IN RESOURCE-LIMITED COUNTRIES

Common MNS disorders include such conditions as mood disorders (e.g., depression and bipolar disorders), anxiety disorders, schizophrenia and other psychotic disorders, obsessive-compulsive disorders, trauma and stressor-related disorders (e.g., post-traumatic stress disorders), dissociative disorders, somatic symptom and related disorders, feeding and eating disorders, substance/medication-induced mental disorders, alcohol-related disorders, tobacco use disorder, and neuro cognitive disorders. Research has shown that they are prevalent globally, including in LMICs [1–3, 18, 19]. They cause much handicap to affected persons through negative effects on their cognition, emotions, behaviour and social functioning. Many times, they present first in primary health care (PHC), but they may be unrecognized and are therefore undertreated.

Moreover, there are not enough mental health specialists to treat these large numbers of patients in different parts of the world [15, 22]. Hence, the World Health Organization (WHO) advocated for a special programme through which non-specialist healthcare providers, working in PHC centres, can recognize and apply the appropriate intervention, be this pharmacological or non-pharmacological. There are many evidence-based interventions available for different types of MNS disorders. Some, such as the innovative 5-Step Patient Interview approach [29], are applied to make the diagnosis of a common mental health condition such as depression easier.

Others, such as cognitive-behavioural therapy (CBT), Integrative Community Therapy (ICT), mindfulness, music therapy, regular walking, spiritual practice, avoiding inappropriate arguments, relaxation therapy, healthy food intake, and narrative therapy are non-pharmacological therapeutic interventions. However, despite the fact that effective methods of treatment abound, only a small proportion of affected persons receive any such treatment, thereby creating a persistent treatment gap, particularly in resource-constrained communities. Many stakeholders (including mental health specialists, health managers, and policymakers, as well as the WHO) are concerned about this and are determined to narrow the gap using a combination of strategies [27, 28].

Globally, there is consensus among researchers, healthcare service managers, and policymakers that the most viable implementation strategy that will deliver optimal mental health care services to those who need them most is to incorporate mental health care services into the general framework of the existing PHC services.

Although efforts have been made by countries to implement this strategy, and some successes have been reported especially in the developed countries, the situation has not been a smooth sail in many LMICs [31, 32]. Implementation has been met with a number of challenges. One recent effort that implemented the mhGAP using non-specialist care providers expectedly recorded much success that was sustained for several months as the proportion of patients who received treatment increased from 0% to 12% for depression, 0% to 8% for alcohol use disorder, 3% to 53% for psychosis, and 1% to 13% for epilepsy [31]. This scenario supports the notion that there already exists many effective evidence-supported interventions to treat mental health conditions globally, including in resource-restricted countries; but sustaining the gains after the implementation is the main impediment. In most countries the same impedances to implementation are encountered at individual, societal, and health system (governmental) levels, and it is evident that any possibility of sustaining closure of the mental health treatment gap in any society or country must address the resistance that will come from these three levels on a long-term basis (Box 6.1).

BOX 6.1 – Seven reasons to integrate mental health care services in primary care

1. The burden of mental disorder is huge.
2. Mental and physical health problems are interwoven.
3. The treatment gap for mental health disorders is enormous.
4. PHC for mental health enhances access.
5. PHC for mental health promotes respect for human life.
6. PHC for mental health is affordable and cost effective.
7. PHC for mental health generates good health outcomes.

Source: WHO/WONCA 2008. 'Integrating mental health into primary care: a global perspective' [30].

A fundamental assumption is often made while desiring to integrate mental health services into primary care – that the existing PHC system is well organised and is functioning optimally. That is, a PHC system that is characterized by transparent, responsible leadership and governance, sustainable financing, a motivated and balanced health workforce, affordable and reliable medicines and vaccines, appropriate information systems, and a responsive service delivery system. Indeed, many countries have been able to achieve PHC status that will assist them to realize provision of universal health coverage [33]. But unfortunately, many PHC systems in most resource-poor countries lack these basic ingredients [32–34]. It is important to address this issue to some extent before attempting to integrate mental health services.

Important factors that serve as barriers to receiving mental care include the population's worldview and cultural belief system with regards to healthcare generally, and mental health specifically.

Stigma and lack of awareness about psychological problems often lead to low perceived need for treatment and the belief that treatment is unlikely to be effective [35]. Individuals and health policymakers in such a society are less likely to be deeply committed to allocating funds and other resources to mental health services.

Financial constraints

Even in the developed world, finance allocated to mental health is still considered as low. But in most LMICs budgetary allocation to mental health care (MHC) is extremely low – some as low as 1% of their total health budget [6]. Hence most individuals in these countries have to fund MHC care by paying out of pocket, further impoverishing them. Although a few countries have funds through taxation and health insurance, very few citizens benefit from these funding measures. Alternative sources of funding are needed to mitigate the crunching effect of medical bills on the majority of patients needing mental care in resource-constrained nations.

Limited workforce and infrastructure

The mental health workforce in all LMICs is grossly inadequate due to limited capacity to produce sufficient numbers of such personnel and the continuous emigration of the few available to other locations that offer them better conditions of service [22–24].

Much research has been conducted on ways to overcome the main challenges and barriers to the integration of mental health into PHC. These include works done to mitigate the impact of stigma and negative cultural attitudes. Investing in ways of improving mental health literacy has been shown to significantly reduce stigma among patients, their families, and even health-care workers [25–27]. Mental health literacy is noted to include the ability to recognize specific disorders; knowing how to seek mental health information; knowing the risk factors and causes, self-treatments, and professional help available; and developing attitudes that promote recognition and appropriate help-seeking [36–38].

Relieving the financial constraints associated with implementing MHC integration is a fundamental necessity. A number of previous workers have made useful suggestions in this regard [39–42]. Most frown at out-of-pocket payment because of its tendency for catastrophic health expenditure. Viable alternatives coming from research in this area include taxation and health care insurance. As recommended by the Lancet Global Health Commission, [42] healthcare financing should be people-centred and should have four distinct attributes: public resources should provide the core of PHC funding; pooled funds should cover PHC; resources should be allocated equitably and protected so they reach frontline providers; and provider payments should be through a blended mechanism with capitation at its core [42].

Shortage of medical workforce is also a major impediment to MHC integration into PHC. But there have been a number of innovative submissions with regard to tackling this problem. It has been strongly recommended that in LMICs non-specialist licensed practitioners (e.g., nurses and pharmacists) should be empowered to perform some of the tasks performed by specialist mental health physicians [43]. But in high-income countries, general practitioners (GPs) are also trained and engaged in providing MHC at the PHC level [44–46]. This may be one major reason why the treatment gap is much lower in those countries. Programme implementers in LMICs should also consider engaging GPs and family physicians[a] much more than is hitherto done [47, 48]. Also, it is advocated that non-licensed healthcare workers such as medical assistants can also be empowered to provide some preventive services by making use of standing orders. In one African country an innovative task-shifting mental health professional category called *psychiatric technicians* was created to serve as a point of entry into the mental health care-provider system [49]. Patients should also be empowered to provide more self-care by harnessing modern technology [50–54]. In the era of COVID-19, mental health care practitioners have also had to lean heavily on telemedicine to deliver psychotherapy and counselling sessions. This trend is likely to persist even after the pandemic [52].

Limited infrastructural capacity

Steps taken to address this problem include training and retraining of available non-specialist personnel on mental health interventions and procedures

[55–59]. When such training is done by mental health specialists it is called task-sharing and this is necessary to ensure that effective interventions and skills are passed on to non-specialist health care providers who will then apply them to patients at the PHC level [55]. They are also expected to scale up these interventions. It has been noted, however, that most of such interventions are hardly sustained let alone scaled up [56, 57]. The mental health training programme must include all cadres of persons that have a stake in mental health care delivery – providers, supervisors, health managers, and policymakers [57, 58]. The ability of the health system to consistently implement the protocols that ensure high-quality care over long periods is possible only when it is supported by high-quality research involving all stakeholders [57, 58].

WHAT SHOULD BE THE PRIORITIES OF THE RESOURCE-CONSTRAINED NATIONS WITH REGARD TO PRIMARY MENTAL HEALTH CARE?

The high burden of MNS disorders in LMICs [1, 2, 9, 10] and the prediction that they are likely to worsen in the near future [17] requires that pragmatic efforts be made to quickly bring them under control. Based on WHO recommendation, and taking a cue from the more developed nations, they should vigorously pursue the integration of mental health services into the general framework of their existing PHC services [59]. This strategy has the potential to reduce stigma, protect patients' rights, improve social integration, reduce chronicity, improve human resource capacity for mental health, and, ultimately, improve access to mental health care [60].

According to the WHO, integrated care is,

> (...) health services that are managed and delivered so that people receive a continuum of health promotion, disease prevention, diagnosis, treatment, disease-management, rehabilitation and palliative care services, coordinated across the different levels and sites of care within and beyond the health sector, and according to their needs throughout the life course.

WHO, 2016, p. 2

In a recent extensive review of the concept, Thornicroft and colleagues [61] showed that, for integrative care to succeed, it must align with the policy priorities of the state or country and must consider the logistical constraints and available resources with the overriding vision to make the provision of mental care an integral component of universal health care provision [61]. Some other necessities include a setting where mental health stigma is minimized through health literacy; a workforce that has the necessary clinical, non-clinical, and emotional skills; a back-up of mental health specialists to provide ongoing training, supervision, and support; and an implementation policy that recognizes the need for collaboration between healthcare and other sectors of the state or nation's life. These ideals in a way define the characteristics of an optimally functioning PHC service [62].

By 2030, mental illness is expected to cost the global community more than US\$6 trillion, taking the impact of mental illness above cardiovascular disease, chronic respiratory disease, cancer, and diabetes [63]. It is known that people with mental illness have a much higher risk of disease and premature death due to physical health issues and their medications than the general population [64]. In these contexts, 75–85% of people with mental health problems go untreated [65]. Combined with a shortage of mental health professionals in LMIC [66], these data point to the importance of primary prevention and interventions at the PHC centre level to improve mental health and well-being. Despite that, mental health problems are inadequately managed in routine practice [67].

INSTRUMENTS AND APPROACHES DEVELOPED IN LMICs

There are instruments and approaches developed in LMICs to help medical and non-medical health professionals to identify and manage psychosocial distress in the population. Next, we will list and comment on some techniques that could be carried out if there were some appropriate training for professionals, for example, 5-Step Patient Interview approach for integrating MHC into PHC services, ICT, music therapy, and mindfulness.

Table 6.1 details non-pharmacological interventions, based on specific mental health cases, and graded in relation to the strength of recommendation and/or certainty of evidence recommended by the WHO and revised in 2023.

5-Step Patient Interview approach for integrating MHC into PHC services

Traditional patient interviews are ineffective in identifying and managing mental health problems in PHC centres [68]. Therefore, the patients' interview process for MHC should be improved to help identify the real problems or issues underlying the complaints [69]. Physicians' skills should be enhanced to empower them to detect and deal with mental health problems and achieve the desired outcomes [70].

TABLE 6.1 Non-pharmacological interventions, based on some conditions, and graded in relation to the strength of recommendation and/or certainty of evidence

Condition	Remark	Strength of recommendation / Certainty of evidence
Alcohol dependence	Network support therapy (including Alcoholics Anonymous attendance) compared with CBT showed an effect for increasing the proportion of days of abstinence.	Moderate certainty
Anxiety	Levels of anxiety in adults with anxiety disorders (GAD or panic disorder) are reduced when engaging in brief, structured psychological interventions based on CBT principles. It can be delivered effectively in non-specialized healthcare settings.	Strong/Moderate
	In resource-constrained settings, stress management techniques (e.g. relaxation training, mindfulness) may be more feasible than psychological interventions, which may require more time and capacity-building.	Conditional/Low
Autism (children and adolescents)	Psychosocial interventions focused on social skills training and developmental behavioural approaches should be offered to improve development, well-being and functioning in children and adolescents with autism.	Strong/Low
	CBT should be offered to children and adolescents with autism with anxiety.	Strong/Moderate
	Organizational skills training focuses on organization of materials, time, and tasks, and includes a variety of learning activities, such as teaching, modelling, and feedback to build new skills or improve performance of existing skills.	Strong/Moderate
Disorders of intellectual development (children)	Beginning-to-read interventions include elements of phonological awareness, letter-sound instruction and decoding.	Strong/Moderate
Cerebral palsy (children and adolescents)	Structured physical exercise and activity should be offered to improve development outcomes, including motor skills and functioning.	Strong/Low
Post-traumatic stress disorder (children and adolescents)	Individual face-to-face CBT with a trauma focus; group face-to-face CBT with a trauma focus; eye movement desensitization and reprocessing (EMDR).	Strong/Moderate

Condition	Intervention	Recommendation
Dementia (carers)	Psychosocial interventions – namely mindfulness-based interventions, multicomponent interventions, psychoeducation and psychotherapy / counselling – should be offered for carers of people living with dementia.	Strong/Low
Dementia (patient)	Physical activity interventions – namely physical exercise delivered 3–4 times per week for 30–45 minutes for more than 12 weeks – should be offered to people living with dementia.	Strong/High
Depression	Structured psychological interventions should be offered for the treatment of adults with moderate-to-severe depression, namely behavioural activation therapy (BAT), brief psychodynamic therapy (DYN), CBT, interpersonal therapy (IPT), problem-solving therapy (PST) and third wave therapies (3WV).	Strong/Moderate
Cocaine and stimulant dependence	CBT and contingency management – should be offered to adults with cocaine and stimulant dependence.	Strong/Low
Psychosis or bipolar disorder (carers)	Problem-solving and cognitive-behavioural approaches (either individual or family-based), self-help interventions and mutual support groups.	Conditional/Moderate
Psychotic disorders (including schizophrenia) in the acute phase	CBT	Conditional/Moderate
Psychosis (including schizophrenia) during the maintenance phase	Family intervention, mindfulness, and CBT	Strong/Moderate

Sources: WHO, 2023; Brohan, Chowdary, Dua et al., 2024.

The 5-Step Patient Interview (AlKhathami approach) is an innovative and concise approach for guiding MHC in PHC centres. It was considered as the first step for implementing the WHO mhGAP Plan 2013–2030. It is proven to be valid and reliable, and has high sensitivity and specificity as compared with expert psychiatrists [29]. Next, the five steps.

Step 1 – Suspicion

This step is the core of this approach. Three patient groups were selected based on a literature review and practical experience. These patients were considered to be more prone to MHC in PHC service.

- *Uncontrolled physical complaints or uncontrolled chronic organic illnesses*: Physical symptoms are more prevalent in patients with depressive and anxiety disorders than in normal subjects [71]. Mental health problems are found to be common among chronic organic ill patients, which have a value impact on the course and outcome of such medical conditions [72].
- *Frequent visits*: Depressed and anxious patients were likely to have unmet patient expectations with doctor shopping and increased provider frustration [73].
- *Sleep disturbance*: Approximately 97% of patients with depression and anxiety experience sleep disturbances [72].

Step 2 – Screening

This step comprises two parts:

- *Hidden agenda and thinking judgement using the idea, concern, expectation (ICE) technique*: The ICE technique is a part of the patient-centred approach [74, 75]. It helps to explore the patient's perception and thinking such as delusions, hallucinations, and flighty ideas, which require immediate referral to a psychiatric clinic.
- *Stress screening (problem's impact) for impact on sleep, performance, and relationships*: Stress screening is a valid and a reliable tool to assess psychological *stress* [29]:
  - *Sleep disturbance*: Early insomnia is considered as an indicator of mild stress presence; interrupted sleep as moderate to severe stress.
  - *Performance and concentration*: An inverse association between performance and psychological stress was found; low performance may indicate the presence of moderate to severe psychological stress [29, 76].

- *Social relationships (isolation and/or easily angered)*: There is a significant association between social isolation, interpersonal sensitivity (low self-esteem), and depression [77]. Moreover, irritability, in which someone is easily angered, is one of the leading indicators of psychological distress that requires careful evaluation. Therefore, when there is a positive tendency for isolation or easy to anger it is an indicator of moderate to severe psychological stress [29].

Step 3 – Service scoping
This step defines where the patient should be served in a PHC centre or psychiatric clinic. Depression and anxiety are the most common mental illnesses and can be managed by PHC doctors [78]. Other psychotic cases can collaborate with mental health specialists for diagnosis and management.

Step 4 – Diagnosis of depression and anxiety
This step applies to PHQ-2 and GAD-2 to diagnose depression and anxiety as recommended [79, 80], in addition to what was mentioned in Steps 1 and 2.

Step 5 – Management
In mild cases, doctors should start the patient on non-pharmacological therapy, including sleep hygiene, regular exercise i.e., walking, deep breath relaxation and supportive therapy. Antidepressant drugs can be initiated if a patient does not respond [78]. For moderate to severe cases, antidepressants should be considered except in two situations:

- *Post-social events*: Narrative therapy should be provided as the first intervention to help patients cope with their problems.
- *Drug side effects on mood*, following administration of drugs such as beta-blockers, contraceptive pills, and steroid medications. In this case, a doctor should modify the medication before considering the antidepressant.

Non-pharmacological therapy:

- *Regular walking*: A meta-analysis showed evidence that walking has wide-ranging health benefits with statistically significant reductions in depression scores [81]. Physical activity affects mood by reducing the activity of the sympathetic nervous system and the associated hypothalamic–pituitary–adrenal axis interaction in the brain [82], which leads to increased levels of both serotonin and norepinephrine in the brain in a manner similar to antidepressant drugs [83]. This improvement is related to the level of cognitive and mood improvement in the brain and behaviour [84]. Six sessions of 20 minutes of treadmill exercise over a two-week period can have a positive effect on mood factors such as anxiety [85]. There are other exercise workouts that have positive effects on mental health problems [86]. Undertaking a 10,000-step walking programme for 100 days ('Happy Feet') also has the effect of improving mental health and well-being [87].

- *Spiritual practice*: Spiritual beliefs and practices appear to play a role as a spiritual coping mechanism to deal with stress [88]. The relationship between religion and mental health ('religion–health connection') has become attractive among therapists as a general protective factor for mental illness [89]. Religious indicators have an impact on mental health outcomes, rates of mood disorders, psychological stress levels, and well-being [90]. Religious participation shows a primary beneficial and protective function in relation to psychological distress, mental health, and well-being outcomes [91]. So, clinicians should consider incorporating spirituality into therapy or at least helping patients use healthy spiritual coping resources as they seek healing [92].
- *Relaxation therapy such as relaxing by deep breathing*: All relaxation exercises such as deep breathing have a positive effect on dealing with stress and promoting well-being [93]. They also have a positive effect by reducing stress, anxiety, and cortisol levels [94].
- *Healthy food intake*: Fruits and vegetables have a positive effect on mental health. Therefore, it is recommended to consume at least five portions of fruits and vegetables daily to help benefit mental health [95].
- *Narrative therapy and CBT*: Research has proven the effectiveness of narrative therapy and CBT in improving mental health states, particularly depression [96].
- *Regular follow-up with a therapist to support improvement*: Regular follow-up with a clinician provides support and augments management improvement.

Figure 6.1 summarizes each step.

Integrative Community Therapy

ICT was created and systematized in the Pirambu favela in the city of Fortaleza in Northeast Brazil, the poorest region in the country, by psychiatrist and anthropologist Adalberto Barreto in 1987. Barreto realized that he could not work in favela communities in the same way he used to work in a hospital setting.

Faced with such a large number of people with psychosocial suffering, many immigrants from the northeastern countryside, he developed a

Step 1 Suspected	Step 2 Screening		Step 3 Scoping	Step 4 Diagnostic	Step 5 Management
Does the patient need MH care?	ICE technique for: • hidden agenda • delusion (if yes, refer to psychiatric)	SPR# (Sleep, Performance, Relationship) for psychological stress screening	Does the patient need Referral?*	Depression (PHQ-2) & or Anxiety (GAD-2)	Antidepressant or only non-pharmacological
Uncontrol medical cases					
Frequent visit	**# SPR technique:** **Sleep** • Early insomnia – mild stress • Interrupted – moderate to severe stress **Performance** • Decline performance – moderate to severe stress **Relationship** • Isolation or easy anger – moderate to severe stress		*** Cases need Referral to psychotic clinics:** - Suicidal thoughts - Postpartum depression - Psychotic symptoms (e.g., hallucinations or delusions) - Childhood psychosis - Personality disorders - Bipolar disorder - Drug abuse - Dementia symptoms - Unresponsive cases		
Sleep disturbance					

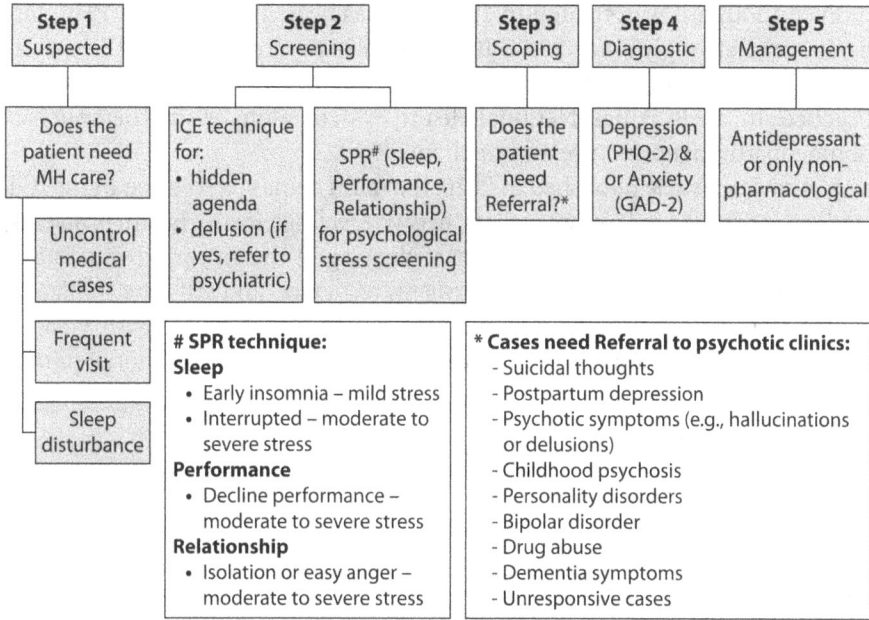

FIGURE 6.1 The 5-Step Patient Interview for mental health care in PHC and family practices (AlKhathami approach, 2022).

method that has as references General System Theory by Von Bertalanffy, Communication Theory by Gregory Bateson, Cultural Anthropology, Pedagogy of the Oppressed by Paulo Freire, and Resilience Theory.

ICT consists of open groups, led by one to three therapists with specific training for this, developing a welcoming space in which it is proposed to listen to suffering and rescue the potential of life stories and community values in order to deal with such situations [97].

According Barreto, the ICT is:

a space for the promotion of interpersonal and inter-community meetings, aiming at valuing the participants' life stories, rescuing their identity, restoring self-esteem and self-confidence, expanding the perception of problems and possibilities for solving them based on local skills. Its support base is the stimulus for the construction of solidarity bonds and the promotion of life.

Barreto, 2008, p. 33 [98]

Even though it was created in 1987 and has been practised in a PHC scenario more strongly since 2004, ICT was incorporated in only 2017 as one of the modalities of the National Policy on Integrative and Complementary Practices in the Brazilian National Health System, along with others such as homoeopathy, acupuncture and medicine [99].

In a review article published in 2020, the main demands received in the ICT circles were related to family conflicts, negative feelings, losses, health problems, and violence. About contributions, participating in the group provided users with autonomy, acceptance, empowerment, resilience, and self-care [100].

ICT that can be used by non-medical health professionals with positive experiences in relation to mental health [101, 102]. Although a large part of the offer is in Brazil, there are ICT services in some Latin American countries and in France [103].

Table 6.2 is a step-by-step for ICT.

TABLE 6.2 The ICT step by step

1. Welcome	• Set the group up. • Putting people at ease and comfortable in a circle. • Community therapist presents what Community Therapy is. • Discussion about the rules
2. Choice of theme	• Speech is open. • Participants present, in a succinct way, the problems or situations that are causing concern. • Everyone chooses the theme and summarily says the reason for the choice.
3. Contextualization	• The person chosen by the group explains the problem or situation presented, with details. • Everyone, including the therapists, can ask questions to further clarify the issue. • The guiding therapist extracts the key question; it is an instrument for transforming the problem from the individual dimension to the group dimension.
4. Problematization	• Everyone responds to the key question, always speaking of their own experience. • The group becomes involved with the problem and the alternatives presented become the group's own.
5. Closure	• An environment of an affective climate is provided; people feel supported by others. • The therapist says positive connotations to everyone who exposed themselves or presented their sufferings. • The therapist asks the participants to talk about the good things that touched and admired them the most. • The session ends with the therapists' thanks and an invitation to the next meetings.

Source: Ref. [98].

Music therapy

Since the second half of the 20th century, there has been a considerable growth of interest in the benefits of cultural participation for health and well-being and, particularly, involvement with the creative arts. Evaluation studies have documented these benefits in a systematic way, contributing to the growth of evidence-based practice [104–106].

In the field of mental health, already in the 1940s, in Brazil, based on the literature of Spinoza, Jung and Artaud, Silveira originally demonstrated the systematic therapeutic effect of spontaneous creative expression in severe mental illness patients, with the creation of the Museum of Images from the Unconscious, the world's largest collection of fine arts produced by mental health patients, still in activity [107].

Empirical studies, most recent in mental health services that offer art as an adjuvant therapeutic tool, point out that involvement in art activities or specially designed art therapies can reduce physical symptoms and improve mental health problems [108–111]. Literature review studies suggest that participatory arts activities and clinical arts interventions are made more widely available in health and social settings [112].

In the field of music therapy in mental health, there is a large historical contribution in the field of practice and production of knowledge [113–116].

Clinical studies provided some evidence that music therapy can be used as an alternative therapy in treating depression, autism, schizophrenia, and dementia, as well as problems of agitation, anxiety, sleeplessness, and substance misuse [117], including studies with adolescents at PHC [118].

Like music, cinema is a powerful instrument of education and adjuvant therapy, even helping medical students to learn and develop competency in the performance of mental status examinations [119, 120].

Digital storytelling process experience, performed by patients and their families, can help to reduce the stigma of mental health, family dynamics and the search for healthcare [121]. In a systematic review, video was found to be more effective than other interventions, such as classical face-to-face educational sessions or simulation of hallucinations. According to the results of two studies, social contact delivered via video achieved a similar destigmatization effect in young people to that delivered via a live intervention [122].

Recently, an Australian documentary series on ABC television, called *Space 22*, proposes artistic interventions in people with mental health problems [123].

Mindfulness

Meditation practices have come to the attention, over at least 50 years, of neuroscientists and psychotherapists. Mindfulness, a meditation practice model, refers to a process of paying attention, on purpose, in the present moment.

As a result, individuals naturally increase their ability to cope with adverse emotional events, generating a great sense of emotional balance and well-being [124, 125].

CMDs, including anxious-depressive syndromes, are being associated with vulnerable social economic conditions such as violence, unemployment, and extreme poverty. CMDs are frequently presented through medically unexplained symptoms, especially pain symptoms, and related to chronic diseases such as hypertension, obesity, and diabetes. They are directly associated with low self-esteem and disempowerment, indirectly associated with a strong social support network, and significantly reduce quality of life.

CMDs are present at large in LMIC, for example, in more than 50% of the total population attending the PHC services in Brazil, especially women [126, 127].

It is necessary, therefore, to offer non-pharmacological treatments, not only psychotherapy and supervised physical activities, but also group interventions as previously presented. The development of group interventions in PHC has been a promising strategy in the care and promotion of mental health, as it develops 'safe spaces' for social inclusion and empowerment, expanding social support networks and increasing the patient's ability to cope with adversity. Among these interventions, mindfulness has proven to be effective in PHC worldwide, both with users and health professionals experiencing burnout [128–130]. In Brazilian PHC, for instance, this cost-effective intervention can offer empowerment and increase in self-esteem, and support from a peer group can help promote well-being and reduce the chronic burden of CMDs [131, 132].

Mental health in rural settings

In rural areas there is usually limited access to care with fewer mental health professionals. The shortage of mental health providers in rural communities requires rural residents to manage a significant time and cost commitment to seek care compared to urban residents [133]. Longer travel times require that rural residents have access to reliable transportation, particularly given that public transportation may not be an option. Rural residents may preferentially rely on social support networks to gain access to these resources, in fact, rural residents have larger social networks and rely more on family members compared to urban residents [134].

Growing concerns about mental health in rural communities

In the United States, there are growing concerns about mental health in rural communities. For example, mental health and mental disorders were the 'most oft-cited priority' by stakeholders for 2030 [135].

Literature suggests that although there is little variability in certain mental health outcomes across the rural–urban continuum, death by suicide is particularly pronounced among rural youth. Evidence suggests that rates of death by suicide are twice as high among rural compared to urban youth and that rural–urban disparities in death by suicide have been widening among boys [136].

Structural barriers impact access to mental health services in rural communities, and these include, for example, a scarcity of mental health providers [137].

Recent studies point to potential differential impacts on mental health between rural and urban areas. While some studies indicate heightened suffering among rural residents, potentially due to limited mental health services or lower socioeconomic status, further analyses presented different findings, suggesting a potentially lower negative impact of the pandemic on mental health in rural areas, possibly attributed to robust social support systems [138–143]. For instance, in France, older adults in rural areas reported better experiences during the first lockdown due to enhanced social support and family presence [143].

Stigma and cultural factors in mental health in rural settings

Mental health issues may carry a significant stigma in rural communities, discouraging individuals from seeking help. Privacy concerns related to seeking mental health services also impact rural residents, particularly rural youth who often rely on their parents to support their health needs.

Specific privacy concerns include worries about stigma and potential social repercussions in small, close-knit communities where confidentiality may be difficult to maintain [144, 145].

Some research on rural–urban differences in stigma has highlighted that stigma is an important issue irrespective of geographic setting but may be particularly relevant for subgroups of rural residents. For example, Shroeder and colleagues found higher levels of stigma regarding mental illness among rural compared to urban women, but no differences between rural and urban men [145]. Stigma seems to be strongest among older generations in a rural community and not being able to seek mental health services anonymously in the small communities discourages mental health help-seeking [137].

Economic factors in mental health in rural settings
Higher poverty rates can limit individuals' ability to pay for care. High poverty rates in rural communities also contribute to disparities in access to mental health care [137].

Missed diagnosis of mental health problems in rural settings

Rural areas do not receive adequate mental health care owing to socioeconomic and geographical reasons and there is ample evidence that primary care physicians have difficulties in diagnosing and treating even common mental disorders such as depression, and psychogeriatric syndromes as well. Even common mental disorders may remain unrecognized in this population and once diagnosed, only a minority of patients receive adequate treatment [146].

Other challenges in providing efficient mental health services in rural areas are difficulties in recruiting, retaining, and developing a trained workforce [147].

Older adults especially may delay or even not contact mental health services for several age-related reasons, such as cognitive decline and physical morbidity, and this may be even more relevant for those living in rural and remote areas, which mostly lack adequate mental health services [146].

Innovations in mental health services in primary healthcare in rural settings – mobile mental health units

To address rural areas' mental health needs, in some countries (Greece), the healthcare system has launched several multidisciplinary teams, the so-called mobile mental health units (MMHUs) [148]. MMHUs are low-cost services because they deliver generic mental health services, and they use the infrastructures and resources of the well-established primary healthcare system in those areas.

These MMHUs which were focused primarily on patients with severe and chronic mental disorders, such as psychotic disorders, treat all referred patients, regardless of diagnosis, as they are the only mental health services in those areas [148].

CONCLUSION

MNS disorders constitute a major disease burden worldwide, but especially in LMICs where more than 80% of affected persons are unable to receive evidence-supported treatments despite these being widely available. This persistent mental health treatment gap in low-resource settings is traceable to the very nature of such nations (low per capita income and widespread poverty, population explosion and high dependency, varying levels of political stability, etc.) and mental health resource-related problems, such as widespread stigma, human resource shortages, reliance on inefficient service delivery models, and low research capacity to reduce the gulf between research and policy implementation of evidence-based interventions.

There is incontrovertible evidence that integration of mental health care into the primary care systems of these countries is the right policy to implement in order to reduce the treatment gap. But such implementation must take into consideration the current level of efficiency of individual countries' PHC system and give preference to interventions that the system can support while at the same time taking all possible measures to strengthen the country's PHC through advocacy involving mental health specialists, primary healthcare managers, health policymakers, and significant others from such sectors as finance, education, legal system, and information technology.

Role of WONCA Working Party on Mental Health

The World Organization of National Colleges, Academies and Academic Associations of General Practitioners/Family Physicians (WONCA) through its Mental Health Consultancies has a major role to play. WONCA (with WHO) may directly engage Ministries of Health in LMICs to offer assistance in terms of workforce training and research capacity-building at the primary-care level. The method of assistance should be country-specific and should be tailored to the current level of efficiency of their PHC systems.

KEY POINTS

- MNS disorders are highly prevalent in low-resource settings, while healthcare delivery in these settings is commonly limited and constrained.
- Effective evidence-based interventions suitable for low resource settings are available.
- What should be the mental health care priorities? What will work? How best to implement?
- Instruments and approaches developed in LMICs.
- Any role for the WWPMH Consultancy group?

---

e-RESOURCES

Implications for primary care practice, including links with community-based approaches:

- http://tinyurl.com/ywmk9dhv
  - The 5-step patient interview (AlKhathami approach)
- https://www.youtube.com/watch?v=RgR9YV0iTIg&ab_channel=MovimentoSa%C3%BAdeMental
  - Integrative Community Therapy (English subtitles)

- http://vivario.org.br/musicoterapia-e-saude-mental-como-a-musica-e-utilizada-no-tratamento-de-pacientes-nos-caps/
  - A music therapist's experience with people with severe mental disorders in a favela in Rio de Janeiro.
- https://www.globalfamilydoctor.com/News/MusicMentalHealthUnveilingPhase2.aspx
  - The Music and Mental Health Project (WONCA Working Party on Mental Health)
- https://u.pcloud.link/publink/show?code=XZl8XrVZdvBsLP1PJUfoJFeCKYpnQLCaoII7
  - Tone of Mind (extended trailer)
- https://mindfulness.unifesp.br/home
  - Brazilian Center for Mindfulness and Health Promotion

NOTE

a In high-income countries usually GPs are post-graduate trained in Family Medicine. In LMICs, generally, the expression GP is related to physicians graduated in medicine, still without any specialization.

REFERENCES

1. Ferrari AJ, Santomauro DF, Mantilla Herrera AMM, et al. Global, regional, and national burden of 12 mental disorders in 204 countries and territories, 1990–2019: a systematic analysis for the Global Burden of Disease Study 2019. Lancet Psychiatry. 2022;9:137–150. doi: 10.1016/S2215-0366(21)00395-3.
2. Steel Z, Marnane C, Iranpour C, et al. The global prevalence of common mental disorders: a systematic review and meta-analysis 1980–2013. Int J Epidemiol. 2014;43(2):476–93. doi: 10.1093/ije/dyu038.
3. World Health Organization. World mental health report: transforming mental health for all. WHO Geneva; 2022. Licence: CC BY-NC-SA 3.0 IGO. Available from: https://www.who.int/publications/i/item/9789240049338. Accessed 10/10/2024.
4. World Health Organization. Global burden of mental disorders and the need for a comprehensive, coordinated response from health and social sectors at the country level [monograph on the internet]. Geneva: WHO; 2012 [cited 2017 Dec 6]. Available from: http://apps.who.int/gb/ebwha/pdf_files/EB130/B130_R8-en.pdf
5. Moitra M, Santomauro D, Collins PY, et al. The global gap in treatment coverage for major depressive disorder in 84 countries from 2000–2019: a systematic review and Bayesian meta-regression analysis. PLoS Med. 2022;19(2):e1003901. doi: 10.1371/journal.pmed.1003901.
6. Rathod S, Pinninti N, Irfan M, et al. Mental health service provision in low-and middle-income countries. Health Serv Insights. 2017;10:1178632917694350. doi: 10.1177/1178632917694350.
7. Kohn R, Ali A, Puac-Polanco V, et al. Mental health in the Americas: an overview of the treatment gap. Rev Panam Salud Publica. 2018;42:e165. doi: 10.26633/RPSP.2018.165.
8. Pan American Health Organization. The Burden of Mental Disorders in the Region of the Americas, 2018. Washington, DC: PAHO; 2018. Available from: https://iris.paho.org/handle/10665.2/49578. Accessed 10/10/2024.
9. Dessauvagie AS, Stein DJ, Jonker D, et al. The prevalence of mental health problems in sub-Saharan adolescents: a systematic review. PLoS ONE. 2021;16(5):e0251689. doi: 10.1371/journal.pone.0251689.

10. Greene MC, Yangchen T, Lehner T, et al. The epidemiology of psychiatric disorders in Africa: a scoping review. The Lancet Psychiatry. 2021;8(8):717–731. doi: 10.1016/s2215-0366(21)00009-2.
11. Funk M, Drew N, Knapp M. Mental health, poverty and development. J Public Mental Health. 2012;11(4):166–185. doi: 10.1108/17465721211289356.
12. Lund C. Poverty, inequality and mental health in low- and middle-income countries: time to expand the research and policy agendas. Epidemiol Psychiatr Sci. 2015;24(2): 97–99. doi: 10.1017/S2045796015000050.
13. International Monetary Fund's World Economic Outlook Database, April 2021. Developing countries 2022. Available from: https://www.imf.org/en/Publications/WEO/weo-database/2022/April. Accessed 10/10/2024.
14. Deepali P. Seven Main Characteristics of Less Developed Countries (LDCs). Available from: https://www.economicsdiscussion.net/economic-growth/7-main-characteristics-of-less-developed-countries-ldcs/14142. Accessed 05/09/2022.
15. Naicker S, Plange-Rhule J, Tutt RC, et al. Shortage of healthcare workers in developing countries–Africa. Ethn Dis. 2009;19(1 Suppl 1):S1–60-4.
16. Bauserman M, Thorsten VR, Nolen TL, et al. Maternal mortality in six low and lower-middle income countries from 2010 to 2018: risk factors and trends. Reprod Health. 2020;17(Suppl 3):173. doi: 10.1186/s12978-020-00990-z.
17. Charlson FJ, Diminic S, Lund C, et al. Mental and substance use disorders in sub-Saharan Africa: predictions of epidemiological changes and mental health workforce requirements for the next 40 years. PLoS ONE. 2014;9(10):e110208. doi: 10.1371/journal.pone.0110208.
18. Naveed S, Waqas A, Chaudhary AMD, et al. Prevalence of common mental disorders in South Asia: a systematic review and meta-regression analysis. Front Psychiatry. 2020;11:573150. doi: 10.3389/fpsyt.2020.573150.
19. Zuberi A, Waqas A, Sadiq N, et al. Prevalence of mental disorders in the WHO Eastern Mediterranean region: a systematic review and meta-analysis. Front Psychiatry. 2021. doi: 10.3389/fpsyt.2021.665019.
20. Demyttenaere K, Bruffaerts R, Posada-Villa J, et al. Prevalence, severity, and unmet need for treatment of mental disorders in the World Health Organization world mental health surveys. JAMA. 2004;291(21):2581–2590. doi: 10.1001/jama.291.21.2581.
21. Asante A, Price J, Hayen A, et al. Equity in health care financing in low- and middle-income countries: a systematic review of evidence from studies using benefit and financing incidence analyses. PLoS One. 2016;11(4):e0152866. doi: 10.1371/journal.pone.0152866.
22. Bruckner TA, Scheffler RM, Shen G, et al. The mental health workforce gap in low- and middle-income countries: a needs-based approach. Bull World Health Organ. 2011;89(3):184–94. doi: 10.2471/BLT.10.082784.
23. Liua JX, Goryakin Y, Maeda A, et al. Global Health Workforce Labor Market Projections for 2030. Policy Research Working Paper; No. 7790. World Bank, Washington, DC. Available from: https://openknowledge.worldbank.org/handle/10986/25035. License: CC BY 3.0 IGO.
24. Michas F. Mental health workforce density by income group 2020. Available from: https://www.statista.com/statistics/452867/density-of-mental-health-workers-by-income-group-of-country. Accessed 10/09/2022.
25. Mubbashar M, Farooq S. Mental health literacy in developing countries. Brit J Psychiatr. 2001;179(1):75. doi: 10.1192/bjp.179.1.75-a.
26. Tambling RR, D'Aniello C, Russell BS, et al. Mental health literacy: a critical target for narrowing racial disparities in behavioral health. Int J Ment Health Addict. 2021:1–15. doi: 10.1007/s11469-021-00694-w.

27. Sweetland AC, Oquendo MA, Sidat M, et al. Closing the mental health gap in low-income settings by building research capacity: perspectives from Mozambique. Ann Glob Health. 2014;80(2):126–133. doi: 10.1016/j.aogh.2014.04.014.

28. AlKhathami AD. An innovative 5-step patient interview approach for integrating mental healthcare into primary care centre services: a validation study. General Psychiatry. 2022;35:e100693. doi: 10.1136/gpsych-2021-100693.

29. World Health Organization/WONCA. Integrating mental health into primary care: a global perspective. Switzerland: World Health Organization; 2008. Available from: https://www.who.int/publications/i/item/9789241563680. Accessed 10/10/2008.

30. Jordans MJD, Luitel NP, Kohrt BA, et al. Community-, facility-, and individual-level outcomes of A district mental healthcare plan in a low-resource setting in Nepal: a population-based evaluation. PLoS Med. 2019;16(2):e1002748. doi: 10.1371/journal.pmed.1002748.

31. Bitton A, Fifield J, Ratcliffe H, et al. Primary healthcare system performance in low-income and middle-income countries: a scoping review of the evidence from 2010 to 2017. BMJ Glob Health. 2019;4(Suppl 8):e001551. doi: 10.1136/bmjgh-2019-001551.

32. Foreign Countries with Universal Health Care. Available from: https://www.health.ny.gov/regulations/hcra/univ_hlth_care.htm. Accessed on 26/10/2022.C

33. Bitton A, Ratcliffe HL, Veillard JH, et al. Primary health care as a foundation for strengthening health systems in low- and middle-income countries. J Gen Intern Med. 2017;32(5):566–571. doi: 10.1007/s11606-016-3898-5.

34. Bresick G, Christians F, Makwero M, et al. Primary health care performance: a scoping review of the current state of measurement in Africa. BMJ Global Health. 2019;4:e001496. doi: 10.1136/bmjgh-2019-001496.

35. Azevedo MJ. The state of health systems in Africa: challenges and opportunities. In: Historical Perspectives on the State of Health and Health Systems in Africa. Palgrave Macmillan, Cham, Volume II. 2017. doi: 10.1007/978-3-319-32564-4_1.

36. Javed A, Lee C, Zakaria H, et al. Reducing the stigma of mental health disorders with a focus on low- and middle-income countries. Asian J Psychiatr. 2021;58:102601. doi: 10.1016/j.ajp.2021.102601.

37. Dang HM, Lam TT, Dao A, et al. Mental health literacy at the public health level in low and middle income countries: an exploratory mixed methods study in Vietnam. PLoS ONE. 2020;15(12):e0244573. doi: 10.1371/journal.pone.0244573.

38. Sweileh WM. Global research activity on mental health literacy. Middle East Curr Psychiatry. 2021;28:43. doi: 10.1186/s43045-021-00125-5.

39. Jorm AF, Korten AE, Jacomb PA, et al. "Mental health literacy": a survey of the public's ability to recognise mental disorders and their beliefs about the effectiveness of treatment. Med J Aust. 1997;166(4):182–186. doi: 10.5694/j.1326-5377.1997.tb140071.x.

40. Abdulmalik J, Olayiwola S, Docrat S, et al. Sustainable financing mechanisms for strengthening mental health systems in Nigeria. Int J Ment Health Syst. 2019;13:38. doi: 10.1186/s13033-019-0293-8.

41. Chisholm D, Docrat S, Abdulmalik J, et al. Mental health financing challenges, opportunities and strategies in low- and middle-income countries: findings from the emerald project - CORRIGENDUM. BJPsych Open. 2021;7(4):e117. doi: 10.1192/bjo.2021.948. Erratum for: BJPsych Open. 2019 Aug 06;5(5):e68.

42. Qin X, Hsieh CR. Understanding and addressing the treatment gap in mental health care: economic perspectives and evidence from China. INQUIRY: The Journal of Health Care Organization, Provision, and Financing. 2020. doi: 10.1177/0046958020950566.

43. Hanson K, Brikci N, Erlangga D, et al. The Lancet Global Health Commission on financing primary health care: putting people at the centre. Lancet Glob Health. 2022;10:e715–e772. doi: 10.1016/S2214-109X(22)00005-5.

44. Sweetland AC, Oquendo MA, Sidat M, et al. Closing the mental health gap in low-income settings by building research capacity: perspectives from Mozambique. Ann Glob Health. 2014;80(2):126–133. doi: 10.1016/j.aogh.2014.04.014.

45. Olfson M. The rise of primary care physicians in the provision of US mental health care. J Health Polit Policy Law. 2016;41(4):559–583. doi: 10.1215/03616878-3620821.

46. Xierali IM, Tong ST, Petterson SM, et al. Family physicians are essential for mental health care delivery. J Am Board Fam Med. 2013;26:114–115. doi: 10.3122/jabfm.2013.02.120219.

47. Cuijpers P, Quero S, Dowrick C, et al. Psychological treatment of depression in primary care: recent developments. Curr Psychiatry Rep. 2019;21(12):129. doi: 10.1007/s11920-019-1117-x.

48. World Health Organization. Primary health care systems (PRIMASYS): case study from Ethiopia, abridged version. Geneva: WHO; 2017. Licence: CC BY-NC-SA 3.0 IGO. Available from: https://iris.who.int/handle/10665/341082. Accessed 10/10/2024.

49. Gureje O, Abdulmalik J, Kola L, et al. Integrating mental health into primary care in Nigeria: report of a demonstration project using the mental health gap action programme intervention guide. BMC Health Serv Res. 2015;15:242. doi: 10.1186/s12913-015-0911-3.

50. Bodenheimer TS, Smith MD. Primary care: proposed solutions to the physician shortage without training more physicians. Health Aff. 2013;32(11):1881–1886. doi: 10.1377/hlthaff.2013.0234.

51. Bhaskar S, Bradley S, Chattu VK, et al. Telemedicine as the new Outpatient Clinic gone digital: position paper from the Pandemic health system REsilience PROGRAM (REPROGRAM) International Consortium (Part 2). Front Public Health. 2020;8:410. doi: 10.3389/fpubh.2020.00410.

52. Chan S, Parish M, Yellowlees P. Telepsychiatry today. Curr Psychiatry Rep. 2015;17(11). doi: 10.1007/s11920-015-0630-9.

53. Fortney JC, Pyne JM, Turner EE, et al. Telepsychiatry integration of mental health services into rural primary care settings. Int Rev Psychiatry. 2015;27(6):525–539. doi: 10.3109/09540261.2015.1085838.

54. Chan S, Godwin H, Gonzalez A, et al. Review of use and integration of mobile apps into psychiatric treatments. Curr Psychiatry Rep. 2017;19:96. doi: 10.1007/s11920-017-0848-9.

55. DeJong SM. Professionalism and technology: competencies across the tele-behavioral health and E-behavioral health spectrum. Acad Psychiatry. 2018;42:800–807. doi: 10.1007/s40596-018-0947-x.

56. Cottler LB, Zunt J, Weiss B, et al. Building global capacity for brain and nervous system disorders research. Nature. 2015;527(7578):S207–S213. doi: 10.1038/nature16037.

57. Ayuso-Mateos JL, Miret M, Lopez-Garcia P, et al. Effective methods for knowledge transfer to strengthen mental health systems in low- and middle-income countries. Br J Psychiatry. 2019;5(5):1–6. doi: 10.1192/bjo.2019.50.

58. Semrau M, Alem A, Abdulmalik J, et al. Developing capacity-building activities for mental health system strengthening in low- and middle-income countries for service users and caregivers, service planners, and researchers. Epidemiol Psychiatr Sci. 2018;27(1):11–21. doi: 10.1017/S2045796017000452.

59. Endale T, Qureshi O, Ryan GK, et al. Barriers and drivers to capacity-building in global mental health projects. Int J Ment Health Syst. 2020;14:89. doi: 10.1186/s13033-020-00420-4.

60. WHO. Sixty-Ninth World Health Assembly, A69/39: Framework on integrated, people-centred health services. Geneva: World Health Organization; 2016. Available from: http://apps.who.int/gb/ebwha/pdf_files/WHA69/A69_39-en.pdf?ua=1&ua=1. Accessed June 7, 2018.

61. Kigozi FN, Ssebunnya J. Integration of mental health into primary health care in Uganda: opportunities and challenges. Ment Health Fam Med. 2009;6(1):37–42.

62. Thornicroft G, Ahuja S, Barber S, et al. Integrated care for people with long-term mental and physical health conditions in low-income and middle-income countries. Lancet Psychiatry. 2018;5(4):456–467. doi: 10.1016/s2215-0366(18)30298-0.

63. Bloom D, Cafiero E, Jané-Llopis E, et al. The global economic burden of noncommunicable diseases. Geneva: World Economic Forum; 2011. REF: 080911. Available from: http://www3.weforum.org/docs/WEF_Harvard_HE_GlobalEconomicBurdenNon CommunicableDiseases_2011.pdf. Accessed 08 October 2024.

64. De Hert M, Correll CU, Bobes J, et al. Physical illness in patients with severe mental disorders. I. Prevalence, impact of medications and disparities in health care. World Psychiatry. 2011;10:52–77. doi: 10.1002/j.2051-5545.2011.tb00014.x.

65. Funk M, Drew N, Knapp M. Mental health, poverty and development. J Public Ment Health. 2012;11:166–185. doi: 10.1108/17465721211289356.

66. Kakuma R, Minas H, van Ginneken N, et al. Human resources for mental health care: current situation and strategies for action. Lancet. 2011;378:1654–1663. doi: 10.1016/S0140-6736(11)61093-3.

67. Read JR, Sharpe L, Modini M, et al. Multimorbidity and depression: a systematic review and meta-analysis. J Affect Disord. 2017;221:36–46. doi: 10.1016/j.jad.2017.06.009.

68. Wagner EH, Austin BT, Von Korff M. Organising care for patients with chronic illness. Milbank Q. 1996;74:511–544.

69. WHO/WONCA. WHO/WONCA Joint Report: Integrating Mental Health into Primary Care - A Global Perspective. WHO Library Cataloguing-in-Publication Data: Singapore; 2008. doi: 10.1080/17571472.2009.11493254. Available from: https://www.tandfonline.com/doi/abs/10.1080/17571472.2009.11493254. Accessed September 2008.

70. Shidhaye R, Lund C, Chisholm D. Closing the treatment gap for mental, neurological and substance use disorders by strengthening existing health care platforms: strategies for delivery and integration of evidence-based interventions. Int J Ment Health Syst. 2015;9:40. doi: 10.1186/s13033-015-0031-9.

71. Bekhuis E, Boschloo L, Rosmalen JG, et al. Differential associations of specific depressive and anxiety disorders with somatic symptoms. J Psychosom Res. 2015;78:116–122. doi: 10.1016/j.jpsychores.2014.11.007.

72. Watson LC, Amick HR, Gaynes BN, et al. Practice-based interventions addressing concomitant depression and chronic medical conditions in the primary care setting: a systematic review and meta-analysis. J Prim Care Community Health. 2013;4:294–306. doi: 10.1177/2150131913484040.

73. AlKhathami AD, Alamin MA, Alqahtani AM, et al. Depression and anxiety among hypertensive and diabetic primary health care patients. Could patients' perception of their diseases control be used as a screening tool? Saudi Med J. 2017;38:621–628. doi: 10.15537/smj.2017.6.17941.

74. Stewart MA, Brown JB, Weston WW, et al. Patient-Centered Medicine: Transforming the Clinical Method. 2nd ed. Oxford-UK: Radcliffe Medical Press; 2003. doi: 10.1111/j.1369-7625.2004.00270.x.

75. Matthys J, Elwyn G, Van Nuland M, et al. Patients' ideas, concerns, and expectations (ICE) in general practice: impact on prescribing. Br J Gen Pract. 2009;59:29–36. doi: 10.3399/bjgp09X394833.

76. Aylaz R, Aktürk Ü, Erci B, et al. Relationship between depression and loneliness in elderly and examination of influential factors. Arch Gerontol Geriatr. 2012;55:548–554. doi: 10.1016/j.archger.2012.03.006.

77. Hirschfeld RM. The comorbidity of major depression and anxiety disorders: recognition and management in primary Care. Prim Care Companion J Clin Psychiatry. 2001;3: 244–254. doi: 10.4088/pcc.v03n0609.

78. WHO. mhGAP Intervention Guide Version 2.0 for mental, neurological and substance use disorders in non-specialised health settings. Geneva: WHO; 2016. Available from: https://www.who.int/publications/i/item/9789241549790. Accessed June 2019.

79. Sapra A, Bhandari P, Sharma S, et al. Using Generalized Anxiety Disorder-2 (GAD-2) and GAD-7 in a primary care setting. Cureus. 2020;12:e8224. doi: 10.7759/cureus.8224.

80. Kroenke K, Spitzer RL, Williams JB. The PHQ-9: validity of a brief depression severity measure. J Gen Intern Med. 2001;16:606–613. doi: 10.1046/j.1525-1497.2001.016009606.x.

81. Hanson S, Jones A. Is there evidence that walking groups have health benefits? A systematic review and meta-analysis. Br J Sports Med. 2015;49(11):710–715. doi: 10.1136/bjsports-2014-094157.

82. Rimmele U, Zellweger BC, Marti B, et al. Trained men show lower cortisol, heart rate and psychological responses to psychosocial stress compared with untrained men. Psychoneuroendocrinology. 2007;32:627–635. doi: 10.1016/j.psyneuen.2007.04.005.

83. Meeusen R, De Meirleir K. Exercise and brain neurotransmission. Sports Med. 1995;20:160–188. doi: 10.2165/00007256-199520030-00004.

84. Szuhany KL, Bugatti M, Otto MW. A meta-analytic review of the effects of exercise on brain-derived neurotrophic factor. J Psychiatr Res. 2015;60:56–64. doi: 10.1016/j.jpsychires.2014.10.003.

85. Smits JAJ, Berry AC, Rosenfield D, et al. Reducing anxiety sensitivity with exercise. Depress Anxiety. 2008;25:689–699. doi: 10.1002/da.20411.

86. Hu S, Tucker L, Wu C, et al. Beneficial effects of exercise on depression and anxiety during the COVID-19 pandemic: a narrative review. Front Psychiatry. 2020;11:587557. doi: 10.3389/fpsyt.2020.587557.

87. Hallam KT, Bilsborough S, de Courten M. "Happy feet": evaluating the benefits of a 100-day 10,000 step challenge on mental health and wellbeing. BMC Psychiatry. 2018;18:19. doi: 10.1186/s12888-018-1609-y.

88. Schuster MA, Stein BD, Jaycox LH, et al. A national survey of stress reactions after the September 11, 2001, terrorist attacks. N Engl J Med. 2001;345:1507–1512. doi: 10.1056/NEJM200111153452024.

89. Ellison CG, Levin JS. The religion-health connection: evidence, theory, and future directions. Health Educ Behav. 1998;25(6):700–720. doi: 10.1177/109019819802500603.

90. Koenig HG, McCullough ME, Larson DB. Handbook of Religion and Health. New York: Oxford University Press; 2001. doi: 10.1093/acprof:oso/9780195118667.001.0001.

91. Levin J. Religion and mental health: theory and research. Int J Appl Psychoanal Stud. 2010;7(2):102–115. doi: 10.1002/aps.240.

92. Koenig HG. Spirituality and mental health. Int J Appl Psychoanal Stud. 2010;7(2):116–122. doi: 10.1002/aps.240.

93. Toussaint L, Nguyen Q, Roettger C, et al. Effectiveness of progressive muscle relaxation, deep breathing, and guided imagery in promoting psychological and physiological states of relaxation. Evid Based Complement Alternat Med. 2021;2021:5924040. doi: 10.1155/2021/5924040.

94. Pardede J, Simanjuntak G, Manalu N. Effectiveness of deep breath relaxation and lavender aromatherapy against preoperative patient anxiety. Divers Equal Health Care. 2020;17(4):168–173.

95. Głąbska D, Guzek D, Groele B, et al. Fruit and vegetable intake and mental health in adults: a systematic review. Nutrients. 2020;12(1):115. doi: 10.3390/nu12010115.

96. Lopes RT, Gonçalves MM, Machado PP, et al. Narrative therapy vs. cognitive-behavioral therapy for moderate depression: empirical evidence from a controlled clinical trial. Psychother Res. 2014;24(6):662–674. doi: 10.1080/10503307.2013.874052.

97. Cisneiros VGF, da Silva Oliveira ML, do Amaral GMDC, et al. Perception of health professionals and community members regarding community therapy in the family health strategy. Rev APS. 2012;15(4). Available from: https://periodicos.ufjf.br/index.php/aps/article/view/14997/7949

98. Barreto ADP. Integrative Community Therapy: Step by Step. 3rd ed. Fortaleza: LCR Press; 2008. doi: 10.4103/WSP.WSP_46_20.

99. Scholze AS, Schwarz TO, de Andrade Reis ML. Community integrative therapy for common mental disorders in primary health care: a systematic review. Rev APS. 2020;23(2). doi: 10.1590/S2237-96222023000100012.

100. Lemes AG, Nascimento VF, Rocha EM, et al. Integrative community therapy in mental health care: an integrative review. Rev Bras Promoç Saúde. 2020;33:10629. doi: 10.5020/18061230.2020.10629.

101. Jatai JM, da Silva LM. Enfermagem e a implantação da Terapia Comunitária Integrativa na Estratégia Saúde da Família: relato de experiência. Rev Bras Enferm. 2012;65(4): 691–695. doi: 10.1590/s0034-71672012000400021.

102. Sena ELDS, Ribeiro DB, Peixoto LCP, et al. Community therapy as a strategy for promoting the mental health of professors in the COVID-19 pandemic. Rev Gaúcha Enferm. 2023;44:e20210133. doi: 10.1590/1983-1447.2023.20210133.en.

103. Abratecom. Associação Brasileira de Terapia Comunitária Integrativa. 2022 [accessed on 2022 Sep 18]. Available from: https://abratecom.org.br/onde-estamos/

104. Helman C. Culture, health and illness. 5th ed. London: Hodder Education; 2007. doi: 10.1201/b13281.

105. Clift S. Arts and health. Perspect Public Health. 2011;131(1):8. doi: 10.1177/1757913911310010401.

106. Sheppard A, Broughton MC. Promoting wellbeing and health through active participation in music and dance: a systematic review. Int J Qual Stud Health Wellbeing. 2020;15(1):1732526. doi: 10.1080/17482631.2020.1732526.

107. Magaldi FS. Psyche meets matter: body and personhood in the medical-scientific project of Nise da Silveira. Hist Cienc Saude Manguinhos. 2018;25:69–88. doi: 10.1590/S0104-59702018000100005.

108. Pordeus V. Restoring the art of healing: a transcultural psychiatry case report. J Psychol Psychother Res. 2014;1(2):47–49. doi: 10.12974/2313-1047.2014.01.02.2.

109. Clift S. Creative arts as a public health resource: moving from practice-based research to evidence-based practice. Perspect Public Health. 2012;132(3):120–127. doi: 10.1177/1757913912442269.

110. Parr H. Mental health, the arts and belongings. Trans Inst Br Geogr. 2006;31(2): 150–166. doi: 10.1111/j.1475-5661.2006.00207.x.

111. Jensen A, Stickley T, Edgley A. The perspectives of people who use mental health services engaging with arts and cultural activities. Ment Health Soc Incl. 2016;20: 180–186. Available from: http://www.emeraldinsight.com/doi/abs/10.1108/MHSI-02-2016-0011

112. Jensen A, Bonde L. The use of arts interventions for mental health and wellbeing in health settings. Perspect Public Health. 2018;138(4):209–214. doi: 10.1177/1757913918772602.

113. Rolvsjord R. Therapy as empowerment: clinical and political implications of empowerment philosophy in mental health practises of music therapy. Nord J Music Ther. 2004;13(2):99–111. doi: 10.1080/08098130409478107.

114. McCaffrey T, Edwards J, Fannon D. Is there a role for music therapy in the recovery approach in mental health? Arts Psychother. 2011;38(3):185–189. doi: 10.1016/j.aip.2011.04.006.

115. Alpert JS. Medicine and music–is there a connection? Am J Med. 2022;135(6):663–664. doi: 10.1016/j.amjmed.2021.11.003.

116. Silverman MJ. Music therapy in mental health for illness management and recovery. Oxford University Press; 2022.

117. Lin ST, Yang P, Lai CY, et al. Mental health implications of music: insight from neuroscientific and clinical studies. Harv Rev Psychiatry. 2011;19(1):34–46. doi: 10.3109/10673229.2011.549769.

118. McFerran KS, Hense C, Koike A, et al. Intentional music use to reduce psychological distress in adolescents accessing primary mental health care. Clin Child Psychol Psychiatry. 2018;23(4):567–581. doi: 10.1177/1359104518767231.

119. Mangot AG, Murthy VS. Cinema: a multimodal and integrative medium for education and therapy. Ann Indian Psychiatry. 2017;1(1):51. doi: 10.4103/aip.aip_13_17.

120. Recupero PR, Rumschlag JS, Rainey SE. The mental status exam at the movies: the use of film in a behavioral medicine course for physician assistants. Acad Psychiatry. 2022;46(3):325–330. doi: 10.1007/s40596-021-01463-6.

121. Otañez M, Lakota W. Digital storytelling: Using videos to increase social wellness. In: Video and Filmmaking as Psychotherapy. Routledge; 2015.

122. Janoušková M, Tušková E, Weissová A, et al. Can video interventions be used to effectively destigmatize mental illness among young people? A systematic review. Eur Psychiatry. 2017;41(1):1–9. doi: 10.1016/j.eurpsy.2016.09.008.

123. ABC's Mental Health Series 'Space 22', Hosted by Natalie Bassingthwaighte, to Air in May. Variety, Australia. 2022 Apr 19. Available from: https://au.variety.com/2022/tv/news/space-22-abc-tv-mental-health-1794/

124. Kabat-Zinn J. Mindfulness-based interventions in context: past, present, and future. Clin Psychol Sci Pract. 2003;10:144–156. doi: 10.1093/clipsy.bpg016.

125. Ludwig DS, Kabat-Zinn J. Mindfulness in medicine. JAMA. 2008;300(11):1350–1352. doi: 10.1001/jama.300.11.1350.

126. Gonçalves DA, Mari JD, Bower P, et al. Brazilian multicentre study of common mental disorders in primary care: rates and related social and demographic factors. Cad Saude Publica. 2014;30(3):623–632. doi: 10.1590/0102-311X00158412.

127. Fortes S, Lopes CS, Villano LAB, et al. Common mental disorders in Petrópolis-RJ: a challenge to integrate mental health into primary care strategies. Braz J Psychiatry. 2011;33(2):150–156. doi: 10.1590/S1516-44462011000200010.

128. Asuero AM, Queraltó JM, Pujol-Ribera E, et al. Effectiveness of a mindfulness education program in primary health care professionals: a pragmatic controlled trial. J Contin Educ Health Prof. 2014;34(1):4–12. doi: 10.1002/chp.21211.

129. Salvado M, Marques DL, Pires IM, et al. Mindfulness-based interventions to reduce burnout in primary healthcare professionals: a systematic review and meta-analysis. Healthcare. 2021;9(10):1342. doi: 10.3390/healthcare9101342.

130. Sundquist J, Palmér K, Johansson LM, et al. The effect of mindfulness group therapy on a broad range of psychiatric symptoms: a randomised controlled trial in primary health care. Eur Psychiatry. 2017;43:19–27. doi: 10.1016/j.eurpsy.2017.01.328.

131. Pizutti LT, Carissimi A, Valdivia LJ, et al. Evaluation of Breathworks' mindfulness for stress 8-week course: effects on depressive symptoms, psychiatric symptoms, affects, self-compassion, and mindfulness facets in Brazilian health professionals. J Clin Psychol. 2019;75(6):970–984. doi: 10.1002/jclp.22749.

132. Demarzo MMP, Andreoni S, Sanches N, et al. Mindfulness-based stress reduction (MBSR) in perceived stress and quality. Health Promot. 2008;14(9):1071–1072. doi: 10.1016/j.explore.2013.12.005.

133. Andrilla CHA, Garberson LA, Patterson DG, et al. Comparing the health workforce provider mix and the distance travelled for mental health services by rural and urban medicare beneficiaries. J Rural Health. 2021;37(4):692–699. doi: 10.1111/jrh.12504.

134. Henning-Smith C, Moscovice I, Kozhimannil K. Differences in social isolation and its relationship to health by rurality. J Rural Health. 2019;35(4):540–549. doi: 10.1111/jrh.12344.

135. Morales DA, Barksdale CL, Beckel-Mitchener AC. A call to action to address rural mental health disparities. J Clin Transl Sci. 2020;4(5):463–467. doi: 10.1017/cts.2020.42.

136. Kreuze E. Mental health and suicide among youth residing in frontier and remote areas. J Clin Psychol. 2024;80(7):1634–1672. doi: 10.1002/jclp.23684.

137. Graves JM, Abshire DA, Koontz E, et al. Identifying challenges and solutions for improving access to mental health services for rural youth: insights from adult community members. Int J Environ Res Public Health. 2024;21(6):725. doi: 10.3390/ijerph21060725.

138. Jia Z, Xu S, Zhang Z, et al. Association between mental health and community support in lockdown communities during the COVID-19 pandemic: evidence from rural China. J Rural Stud. 2021;82:87–97. doi: 10.1016/j.jrurstud.2021.01.015.

139. Monnat SM. Rural-urban variation in COVID-19 experiences and impacts among US working-age adults. Ann Am Acad Pol Soc Sci. 2021;698(1):111–136. doi: 10.1177/00027162211069717.

140. Desdiani D, Sutarto AP. Impact of the restrictions on community activities policy during the COVID-19 on psychological health in Indonesia's urban and rural residents: a cross-sectional study. Health Sci Rep. 2022;5(5):e725. doi: 10.1002/hsr2.725.

141. Henning-Smith C, Meltzer G, Kobayashi LC, et al. Rural/urban differences in mental health and social well-being among older US adults in the early months of the COVID-19 pandemic. Aging Ment Health. 2023;27(3):505–511. doi: 10.1080/13607863.2022.2060184.

142. Liu L, Xue P, Li SX, et al. Urban-rural disparities in mental health problems related to COVID-19 in China. Gen Hosp Psychiatry. 2021;69:119. doi: 10.1016/j.genhosppsych.2020.07.011.

143. Pérès K, Ouvrard C, Koleck M, et al. Living in rural area: a protective factor for a negative experience of the lockdown and the COVID-19 crisis in the oldest old population? Int J Geriatr Psychiatry. 2021;36(12):1950–1958. doi: 10.1002/gps.5609.

144. Ferris-Day P, Hoare K, Wilson RL, et al. An integrated review of the barriers and facilitators for accessing and engaging with mental health in a rural setting. Int J Ment Health Nurs. 2021;30(6):1525–1538. doi: 10.1111/inm.12929.

145. Schroeder S, Tan CM, Urlacher B, et al. The role of rural and urban geography and gender in community stigma around mental illness. Health Educ Behav. 2021;48(1):63–73. doi: 10.1177/1090198120974963.

146. Peritogiannis V, Lixouriotis C. Mental health care delivery for older adults in rural Greece: unmet needs. J Neurosci Rural Pract. 2019;10(4):721–724. doi: 10.1055/s-0039-3399603.

147. Palomin A, Takishima-Lacasa J, Selby-Nelson E, et al. Challenges and ethical implications in rural community mental health: the role of mental health providers. Community Ment Health J. 2023;59(8):1442–1451. doi: 10.1007/s10597-023-01151-9.

148. Peritogiannis V, Fragouli-Sakellaropoulou A, Stavrogiannopoulos M, et al. The role of the Mobile Mental Health Units in Mental Healthcare delivery in rural areas in Greece: current challenges and prospects. Psychiatriki. 2022;33(4):301–309. doi: 10.22365/jpsych.2022.084.

149. World Health Organization. Mental Health Gap Action Programme (mhGAP) guideline for mental, neurological and substance use disorders [Internet]. 2023. Available from: https://iris.who.int/bitstream/handle/10665/374250/9789240084278-eng.pdf?sequence=1.

150. Brohan E, Chowdhary N, Dua T, et al. The WHO mental health gap action programme for mental, neurological, and substance use conditions: the new and updated guideline recommendations. Lancet Psychiatry. 2024;11(2):155–158. doi: 10.1016/S2215-0366(23)00370-X.

CHAPTER 7

Improving interface between generalists and psychiatrists

Abdullah Dukhail AlKhathami
and Ana B. Pérez Villalva

INTRODUCTION

Joseph is 56. He lives with his wife Sharon and three children, two of them minors. He visits his family doctor every three months as part of his follow-up due to a previous diagnosis of diabetes mellitus, which has remained under control for the last six months. In the last month he went to the emergency room due to the presence of diabetic ketoacidosis: his laboratory studies have been altered, with elevations in fasting capillary glucose. He appears sad during the consultation. He speaks little. His wife reports that he has had mood swings, he sleeps more hours, and no longer shows joy in activities that she believes he was passionate about before. During the consultation Joseph states that he was fired last month and that he has not been able to find a new job.

Mental health problems are commonly encountered in primary care centres, with a prevalence of 60% [1]. Depression and anxiety are the most common causes of these problems. Wittchen et al. estimated that at least 50% of the population experience mental health problems throughout their lives [2]. In addition, at least one-third of consultations in primary care have a direct and explicit psychological component. According to the Pan American Health Organization [3], 75–90% of people who suffer from mental health problems do not receive the treatment they need, even though effective treatment is available. This has created a gap in mental health care.

DOI: 10.1201/9781003473947-10

The Mental Health Gap Action Programme (mhGAP) aims to address the unmet needs of people with mental, neurological, and substance-use conditions in non-specialized health services [3]. The characteristics of the new mental health model are comprehensive, integrated, accessible, and high quality, with a health services network approach. Its principles are universal healthcare coverage, evidence-based practices, person-centred and life-course care, multisectoral approach, and empowerment. Although the demand for mental health care treatment has been increasing, studies have demonstrated a shortage of mental health care clinicians and limited access to mental health care [4].

CHALLENGES IN IMPLEMENTING mhGAP IN PRIMARY CARE CENTRES

PHC is under increasing pressure, especially when it is perceived that many consultations are undertaken under the pressure of productivity assessment based on the time and number of consultations given. This is important when considering that identified barriers include a lack of time, skills, and training needed to deal with mental health problems [5]. Mental health problems are among the most common and expensive conditions [6]. Untreated mental illnesses are associated with decreased functionality, reduced quality of life, increased physical health complications, and premature mortality [7].

Therefore, the interest in conducting several trials to implement the mhGAP programme since its launch in 2010, and its revision as a second edition in 2016, has been towards primary mental health care that treats low- and moderate-risk mental health care conditions in PHC [8]. However, serious psychiatric cases are referred to a mental health care specialist. According to the World Health Organization (WHO), integrating mental health services into primary care is the most feasible way to close the treatment gap and ensure that people get the mental health care they need. Aso, there is a huge gap in care for the most common mental health cases such as depression and anxiety, so countries must find innovative ways to diversify and expand the scope of care for these conditions [9]. Therefore, PHC providers play a critical role in meeting the mental health needs of many patients because they are the first line of contact for these patients.

A literature review done by Wakida et al. [10] demonstrated that the policy of integrating mental health into PHC has been implemented in different countries, but there is still weak or no integration in service delivery. One of the important factors that must be taken into consideration for success is the adoption of policies in those countries to support service providers in PHC centres with training and job description that allow them to provide primary mental health care within their daily work. It is worth noting that financial resources were not an obstacle, but rather a facilitating factor.

Despite the existence of training and qualification protocols and manuals of sufficient quality, the desired goals have not yet been achieved. Adopting the patient interview approach used in specialized mental health clinics to train family doctors and PHC workers is considered the most prominent obstacle and barrier to the success of the integration process.

While the main defect is not the inability to diagnose or deal with mental disorders, the problem has three important factors that must be considered to bridge the gap at the PHC centre level:

- *Setting*: PHC centres are usually crowded with patients, as the time available to meet patients is much less than that available in a specialized psychiatric clinic.
- *Healthcare provider*: The family and PHC centre doctors serve all specialties, not just psychological disorder specialists. Therefore, dealing with a physical illness is easier and faster than dealing with a psychological illness, which requires a longer time and broader discussion.
- *Illness symptoms*: Organic diseases are characterised by well-known and specific symptoms and signs that are easy to recognize and diagnose. Patients with mental disorders and illnesses often present with uncontrolled physical symptoms and complaints. This leads to mental health problems that are not discovered or are incorrectly diagnosed. Such an approach increases the patient's suffering, diagnostic tests, and rumours to reach the cause of the disease, as it is an organic disease. In addition, medications are prescribed, and doses are increased to unsuccessfully control the symptoms.

BRIDGING THE MENTAL HEALTH CARE GAP AT THE PHC LEVEL

It is important to find an approach to interviewing patients that is appropriate for the situation in PHC and to consider the previously mentioned factors that played a role in not achieving the goals of integrating mental health into PHC. Recently, an innovative approach called the 'Five-Step Patient Interview for the Provision of Primary Mental Health Care in Primary Care Centres' has been created that enables PHC doctors to provide mental health care services within their daily work [11]. This is a concise, modern, and highly effective approach compared with the work of psychiatric experts and the PHQ-9 and GAD-7. This allows mental health care services to be integrated into doctors' work in a short time, averaging 4.2 minutes. It also professionally defines the roles of PHC and mental health care professionals. It aims to increase doctors' efficiency in managing depression and anxiety. Patients with other mental disorders are referred to a specialist using a referral system.

Models of collaboration between family medicine and mental health specialists for providing mental health care in PHC

PHC providers play a crucial role in addressing patients' mental health needs and providing access to care [1]. However, the shortage of specialist availability represents a growing need for timely specialist advice and increased collaboration between generalists and psychiatrists to reduce gaps in care [12]. It has been demonstrated that family and primary care doctors must collaborate with psychiatric specialists in order to provide effective services. In addition, encouraging effective communication in order to provide better care for mental health patients in PHC settings [13].

Thus, the collaborative model allows generalists better access to mental health specialists, serves as a bridge to improve timely access to specialist opinions, and supports generalists in delivering mental health care [14]. The opportunity for collaboration between a generalist and psychiatrist can be achieved through various models, as follows.

Expanding the role of family doctors in mental health

The involvement of family doctors in monitoring mental health pathologies goes beyond mere diagnosis; it incorporates the vital task of longitudinal care. This approach ensures that patients receive continuous support, which is often critical in chronic mental health conditions. A review of studies on family doctors' roles in mental health care has demonstrated that their understanding of patients' life contexts significantly enhances the quality of care [5]. Evidence shows that patients who establish trusting relationships with their primary care providers report higher satisfaction and adherence to treatment plans [15].

Additionally, family doctors are uniquely positioned to address the stigma surrounding mental health. A study by Thornicroft et al. [16] revealed that stigma reduction in medical settings significantly increases patients' willingness to seek help. Educating patients and their families about mental health as part of regular consultations can dismantle harmful stereotypes and encourage open conversations.

Advantages of community-oriented care

Community-based care, facilitated by family doctors, is crucial in regions where psychiatric resources are limited. In Latin America, for instance, integrated models where primary care physicians take on mental health responsibilities have proven effective [17]. According to a case study in Brazil, integrating mental health care into PHC settings led to a 25% reduction in depressive symptoms among patients after one year [18]. Such models demonstrate the value of leveraging local resources to provide accessible care.

The integration of family dynamics into treatment plans aligns with the biopsychosocial model of health, which emphasizes the interplay between biological, psychological, and social factors. Family doctors' ability to engage with patients on all three levels ensures a holistic approach to care, improving outcomes for mental health conditions that are often exacerbated by social stressors [19].

Reducing barriers to care

Breaking down barriers to mental health care involves both systemic- and individual-level interventions. At the systemic level, the adoption of policies that prioritize mental health integration into PHC settings is essential. A global survey by the WHO [9] found that countries with robust mental health integration policies reported better outcomes in terms of accessibility and patient satisfaction.

On an individual level, family doctors can employ patient-centred approaches, including motivational interviewing and culturally sensitive care. Evidence from a randomized controlled trial in the United States demonstrated that motivational interviewing significantly improves adherence to treatment plans among patients with depression and anxiety [20]. Additionally, tailoring interventions to align with patients' cultural backgrounds enhances their relevance and efficacy [21].

STRENGTHENING EVIDENCE-BASED PRACTICES

To further strengthen the argument, incorporating evidence-based practices into the discussion is critical. For example:

- *Psychosocial Interventions*: Studies have shown that incorporating activities such as mindfulness meditation and structured recreational programmes into care plans reduces anxiety and depression scores [22].
- *Interdisciplinary Collaboration*: A systematic review highlighted that collaborative care models, which include mental health specialists and generalists working together, improve patient outcomes and reduce healthcare costs [23].

SHARED CARE

It is important to improve patient care rather than to segment care between sectors. However, there is no evidence that segmentation of care will reduce activity in either sector or offer opportunities for cost containment [24].

Theoretically, shared care represents an opportunity for patients to receive the benefits of specialist intervention alongside the continuity of care and comorbidity management provided by generalists. General practitioners and family physicians are responsible for all aspects of a patient's healthcare, including the diagnosis, treatment, and follow-up of chronic diseases, with enhanced information exchange and reliable referral when needed. Family physicians with access to collaborative care report greater knowledge, better skills, greater comfort in managing psychiatric disorders, and greater satisfaction with mental health services [25].

a. *Psychiatric e-Consults*: e-Consults are provider-to-provider communications within shared electronic medical records or web-based platforms. Thus, the use of e-Consults has steadily expanded over the years, serving as an opportunity to improve healthcare quality and reduce specialty care costs [26, 27].

b. *Liaison*: A liaison meeting is attended by specialists and primary care team members who discuss and plan the ongoing treatment of patients within the service.

c. *Basic model*: A specific and regular communication system has been established between specialties and primary care. This may be enhanced by an administrator who organises appointments, follows up, and recalls defaulters from care.

d. *Shared care record card*: In a more formal arrangement for information sharing, an agreed upon dataset is entered onto a record card that is usually carried by the patient.

THERAPEUTIC PLAN FOR JOSEPH

In the case of Joseph, who we introduced at the beginning of this chapter, we now describe his therapeutic plan.

During the consultation, some open and circular questions are asked that obtain some family patterns related to Joseph's emotional behaviour. In addition, a genogram is carried out through which the patterns of relationships between family members are considered. Within the interview, a count is also made of the resources that the patient has. Alarm data are questioned, the patient does not present any. Sharon, his wife, also mentions that two weeks ago they decided to go to a consultation with a psychiatrist who began pharmacological treatment. However, Joseph expresses some doubts and fears that these medications are what are causing his current state of lack of control in his chronic degenerative pathology.

The doubts that the patient has are clarified, especially regarding the average duration of treatment and the appearance of adverse effects. He mentions that, given the relationship that his family has had with the family doctor, he trusts the answers of his family doctor and wanted to make sure that what was indicated by the other doctor was appropriate. In this same consultation he is referred to nutrition as part of his treatment, modifications are made to his pharmacological treatment for diabetes mellitus, and new laboratory studies are indicated for his next consultation in a month. He is scheduled for a consultation in two weeks for exploratory purposes and to begin non-pharmacological treatments.

In the next consultation, Joseph is more open to talking about the factors surrounding his emotional state. An integrative exercise is conducted using a table to assess and consolidate the patient's available resources across multiple domains. These include family support, religious affiliation (with regular practice of Buddhism), and economic resources–with plans in place to provide guidance through social work to help the patient access government assistance while seeking new employment. The patient's educational background is also a valuable asset, as he holds postgraduate qualifications. In terms of social support, he maintains strong connections with friends and neighbours. Recreationally, he remains active and engaged: he plays soccer every Saturday, frequently goes to the movies, has attended painting classes, and enjoys woodworking and carpentry in his free time. According to his wife, he has stopped doing several of these activities. He says that, before, they went out to dinner together at least once a week and watched at least one movie together a week. It is discussed with them that it is important to resume at least one of these two activities, which will encourage dialogue and the expression of emotions. Especially since they have argued too much recently, and Sharon has reconsidered temporarily separating from Joseph.

It is evident during the consultation that they maintain language distortions, many generalisations are seen in their speech, they use 'always' and 'never' in their conversation. In this consultation, referral to medical family therapy is suggested, to ensure that communication improves, that it is direct and effective, that they can understand each other and that they maintain a space where they can practise making more favourable interactions. Communication is maintained with the therapist to whom it is sent, to jointly define the objectives to be achieved. In addition, a telephone call is obtained with the psychiatrist to include him in the planning of objectives and in the evaluation of their scope.

Joseph continues to keep his follow-up appointments every month. In the following three months, he shows progress in his physical, emotional, psychological, and mental state. He has taken on the task of finding a new job; he says he has two interviews scheduled that same week. He has started gardening with Sharon. Additionally, once a week, they go to a Buddhist centre. They practise meditation together daily. In therapy they have decided to go for a walk through the city once a month, alone, without their children. This has allowed them not only to improve their communication, but also understanding and greater ease in expressing their emotions. He has lost weight, and he implemented a diet again. His laboratory studies have come out within normal parameters, and he says he feels optimistic about the future.

Joseph's progress has been achieved through the collaborative work carried out with the entire team involved in its management. Effective and efficient communication between members of the health teams guarantees that the objectives remain achievable and that they can be evaluated from different perspectives.

RECOMMENDATIONS

To improve the interface between generalists and psychiatrists, and bridge the mental health care gap in PHC, the following recommendations are proposed:

1. **Strengthen Training and Skill Development**
   - *Mandatory Training for PHC Providers*: Incorporate comprehensive training on mental health conditions, focusing on early detection, treatment, and referral pathways. Programs like the mhGAP should be adapted to local needs.
   - *Continuing Education*: Offer regular workshops and refresher courses to ensure generalists stay updated on mental health advancements, evidence-based practices, and culturally sensitive approaches.

2. **Promote Collaborative Care Models**
   - *Shared Care Models*: Develop and implement shared care frameworks where generalists and psychiatrists work in tandem to manage patient care, ensuring continuity and integration of services.
   - *Psychiatric e-Consultation Systems*: Expand the use of e-Consult platforms to facilitate timely access to specialist opinions, particularly in resource-limited settings.

3. **Enhance Communication Channels**
   - *Regular Liaison Meetings*: Establish structured meetings between PHC teams and psychiatrists to discuss and plan ongoing patient care collaboratively.
   - *Shared Medical Records*: Implement interoperable systems for seamless communication and shared decision-making among healthcare providers.

4. **Integrate Community-Based Interventions**
   - *Leverage Local Resources*: Train family doctors to use community resources such as religious groups, educational programmes, and social networks to support patients with mental health conditions.
   - *Stigma-Reduction Campaigns*: Engage community leaders, patients, and families in awareness programmes to address stigma and promote acceptance of mental health care.

5. **Adopt Patient-Centred Interview Approaches**
   - *Five-Step Patient Interview*: Encourage the adoption of concise and effective interview methods, such as AlKhathami's Five-Step approach, to improve the efficiency and quality of mental health care in PHC.
   - *Motivational Interviewing*: Train providers in techniques to enhance patient engagement, address ambivalence, and improve treatment adherence.

6. **Policy and Infrastructure Development**
   - *Supportive Policies*: Advocate for policies that prioritise mental health integration into PHC, ensuring adequate resources, time, and staffing for mental health care.
   - *Infrastructure Investments*: Strengthen PHC centres with the necessary tools, privacy provisions, and staffing to manage mental health conditions effectively.

7. **Monitor and Evaluate Outcomes**
   - *Quality Metrics*: Develop and track key performance indicators (KPIs) to evaluate the success of integration efforts, such as improved patient satisfaction, reduced referral rates, and better clinical outcomes.
   - *Feedback Mechanisms*: Incorporate patient and provider feedback to refine collaborative care models and address barriers to effective mental health care delivery.

8. **Scale Up Community Clinics**
   - *Specialist Presence in PHC Settings*: Encourage psychiatrists to provide regular services within PHC clinics to foster informal and trust-based communication with generalists.
   - *Focus on Family Dynamics*: Equip family doctors with tools to assess and address family dynamics that may influence mental health outcomes, enhancing their holistic approach.

These recommendations aim to create robust, integrated, and sustainable mental health care.

REFERENCES

1. WHO – *Integrating Mental Health into Primary Care: A Global Perspective* (PDF). 2008. https://iris.who.int/bitstream/handle/10665/43935/9789241563680_eng.pdf
2. Wittchen HU, Mühlig S, Beesdo K. Mental disorders in primary care. Dialogues Clin Neurosci. 2003;5(2):115–128.
3. Pan American Health Organization. Mental Health in Primary Care. 2025. https://www.paho.org/en/topics/mental-health-primary-care
4. Thomas KC, Ellis AR, Konrad TR, Holzer CE, Morrissey JP. County-level estimates of mental health professional shortage in the United States. Psychiatr Serv. 2009;60(10):1323–1328.
5. Brown M, Moore CA, MacGregor J, Lucey JR. Primary care and mental health: overview of integrated care models. J Nurse Pract. 2021;17(1):10–14.
6. Roehrig C. Mental disorders top the list of the most costly conditions in the United States: $201 billion. Health Aff (Millwood). 2016;35(6):1130–1135.
7. Fagiolini A, Goracci A. The effects of undertreated chronic medical illnesses in patients with severe mental disorders. J Clin Psychiatry. 2009;70(Suppl 3):22–29.
8. World Health Organization. mhGAP programme version 2.0. mhGAP Intervention Guide for mental, neurological and substance use disorders in non-specialized health settings. Version 2.0. 2016. https://www.who.int/europe/publications/i/item/9789241549790
9. World Health Organization. Mental health: strengthening our response [Internet]. Geneva: World Health Organization. 2022. http://www.who.int/features/factfiles/mental_health/en/
10. Wakida EK, Talib ZM, Akena D, Okello ES, Kinengyere A, Mindra A, Obua C. Barriers and facilitators to the integration of mental health services into primary health care: a systematic review. Syst Rev. 2018;7(1):211
11. AlKhathami AD. An innovative 5-Step patient interview approach for integrating mental healthcare into primary care centre services: a validation study. Gen Psychiatry. 2022;35:e100693.
12. World Health Organization. Mental health integration in primary care: Global perspectives and lessons learned. Geneva: WHO, 2018.
13. Althubaiti N, Ghamri R. Family physicians' approaches to mental health care and collaboration with psychiatrists. Cureus. 2019;11(5):e4755.
14. Kukafka R, Avery J, Dwan D, Sowden G, Duncan MD. Primary care psychiatry eConsults at a rural academic medical center: descriptive analysis. J Med Internet Res. 2021;23(9):e24650.
15. Mitchell ED, Rubin G, Macleod U. The role of primary care in cancer diagnosis via emergency presentation: qualitative synthesis of significant event reports. BJGP Open. 2019;3(4). https://bjgpopen.org/content/3/4/bjgpopen19X101670.short
16. Thornicroft G, Mehta N, Clement S, et al. Evidence for effective interventions to reduce mental-health-related stigma and discrimination. Lancet. 2020;387(10023):1123–1132.
17. Ángel M. Fortalecimiento de la salud mental en México: recomendaciones para una psiquiatría comunitaria. Salud Ment. 2016;39(4):235–237.
18. da Silva M, Loureiro S, Crippa J. Mental health integration in primary care: a case study in Brazil. J Integr Care. 2020;28(3):267–280.
19. Balasubramanian S, Anand AK, Sawant PS, Rao BC, Prasad R. Managing mental health problems in a family and community setting: reflections on the family physician approach and Re-imagining psychiatric education. J Family Med Prim Care. 2021;10(4):1639–1643. https://doi.org/10.1038/bjc.2015.42
20. Miller WR, Rollnick S. Motivational Interviewing: Helping People Change. Guilford Press, 2013.

21. Bhugra D, Becker M. Migration, cultural bereavement and cultural identity. World Psychiatry, 2005;4(1):18–24.

22. Goyal M, Singh S, Sibinga E, et al. Meditation programs for psychological stress and well-being: a systematic review and meta-analysis. JAMA Internal Medicine. 2014;174(3):357–368.

23. Woltmann E, Grogan-Kaylor A, Perron B, et al. Comparative effectiveness of collaborative chronic care models for mental health conditions across primary, specialty, and behavioral health care settings: systematic review and meta-analysis. Am J Psychiatry. 2012;169(8):790–804.

24. Smith SM, Cousins G, Clyne B, Allwright S, O'Dowd T. Shared care across the interface between primary and specialty care in management of long-term conditions. Cochrane Database Syst Rev. 2017;2(2):CD004910.

25. Kisely S, Duerden D, Shaddick S, Jayabarathan A. Collaboration between primary care and psychiatric services: does it help family physicians? Can Fam Physician. 2006;52:876–877.

26. Liddy C, Afkham A, Drosinis P, Joschko J, Keely E. Impact of and satisfaction with a new eConsult service: a mixed methods study of primary care providers. J Am Board Fam Med. 2015;28(3):394–403.

27. Archibald D, Stratton J, Liddy C, Grant RE, Green D, Keely EJ. Evaluation of an electronic consultation service in psychiatry for primary care providers. BMC Psychiatry. 2018;18(1):119.

SECTION 3

CHAPTER 8

End of life

The new paradigm that has been developed in response to COVID-19 with a focus on home and palliative care

James Jackson, Christos Lionis, and Juan Mendive

PRIMARY PALLIATIVE CARE

The World Health Assembly resolved that palliative care is 'an ethical responsibility of health systems' and that integration of palliative care into public health care systems is essential for the achievement of the Sustainable Development Goal on universal health coverage.[1] A comprehensive guideline was published in 2018 as a result, where the World Health Organization (WHO) advocated for integrating palliative care into primary care.[2]

Palliative care is a sub-specialization of medicine focused on supporting patients with serious and complex illnesses with the aim of optimizing quality of life, mitigating suffering, and guiding plans of care around goals and values. Primary palliative care refers to the foundational skills and practices of palliative care that are considered core competencies of any medical provider (family physicians as well as specialty providers like oncologists). Primary palliative care includes symptom management (pain, nausea, etc.) as well as communication skills.

Symptom management in primary palliative care includes non-pharmacological and pharmacological treatment, including opioids. Opioid use in symptom management varies widely around the world due to stigma,

DOI: 10.1201/9781003473947-12

access, and law. As a result, training and comfort with these medications is almost universally inadequate. Digitalization of resources for medical providers has expanded access to evidence-based references for symptom management. The Pink Book[3] is an open-access resource maintained by an interdisciplinary team of palliative care experts at the Dana Farber Cancer Institute in Boston, Massachusetts. Fast Facts[4] is another valuable open resource managed by the Palliative Care Network of Wisconsin and provides a wider range of information relevant to primary care physicians.

Communication comprises the other major skill set in primary palliative care, outside of symptom management, and goes beyond 'bedside manner'. Communication skills are increasingly being taught in the same way as procedural skills. Palliative care communication is often pigeonholed as a way to break bad news. While breaking bad news is certainly an important communication skill, palliative care communication really aims to understand patient/family goals and values in balance with medical reality and expertise to guide care planning and recommendations. This can be done through a 'serious illness conversation'. The REMAP[5] framework and SIC[6] (serious illness conversation) Guide are two frameworks for this fundamental skill in primary palliative care. The serious illness conversation follows a stepwise progression that starts from illness understanding and ends with recommendations/plan for next steps. Just like procedural training, communication skills in primary palliative care *can* be taught and practice is key. Communication skills not only strengthen trust and provide support to patients/families, but also save time by having deliberate, effective communication rather than frequent, often repetitive, ineffective communication. Taking time in a conversation to allow for silence, respond to emotion, demonstrate understanding, and align with patient goals/values is summed up in the palliative care mantra – 'go slow to go fast.'

While primary palliative care skills are essential for family physicians, access to advanced palliative care is critical for health systems to operate effectively. However, many parts of the world do not have access to palliative care. Alongside the 'mental health care gap', the 'global suffering gap' – which represents the discrepancy in need for palliative care and access to palliative care – is only getting wider as non-communicable diseases (NCDs) become more burdensome, especially in low- and middle-income countries (LMICs). As the WHO works to address the need for mental health care with mhGAP (Mental Health Gap Action Programme), there is growing recognition of the need for palliative care both at the individual and at the systems level. Just as with mental health, palliative care not only improves the lives of individuals and families, but also provides a cost savings for healthcare systems when considering disability-adjusted life years (DALYs) and end-of-life medical care costs. Many nations are working at the ministry level to improve access to critical medications like morphine and are investing to embed palliative care in oncology care. At the same time, grass-roots efforts in primary palliative care are innovating solutions through collaborative care models, learning networks, and global partnerships.

ADDRESSING MENTAL HEALTH IN PRIMARY PALLIATIVE CARE

Living with or caregiving for people with serious illness is a significant risk factor for mental illness. Common psychiatric disorders in people experiencing (directly or indirectly) the stress of serious illness can include depression, anxiety, adjustment disorder, post-traumatic stress disorder (PTSD), and grief disorder. In fact, a whole sub-specialty of psycho-oncology exists to better address the mental health needs in patients with cancer. In primary care settings, though, it can feel unclear to diagnose mental illness in this population where special care is taken not to over pathologize the continuum of normal distress. Moreover, the high degree of overlap of diagnostic criteria can lead to uncertainty and hesitancy to recommend any treatments. With both the DSM-5 and the ICD-11, there has been an intentional movement thinking about diagnoses as each representing a distinct pathology towards understanding symptoms as features on a broader diagnostic spectrum. In the global health domain, where focus tends to be more on population-based implementation and outcome measures, there has been a lot of interest in a new approach to mental health in primary care – the transdiagnostic approach.[7]

The transdiagnostic approach aims to optimize function through earlier management (both psychotherapy and psychopharmacology) where there is treatment convergence along the differential diagnoses. Example: a 50-year-old man was diagnosed three weeks ago with metastatic pancreatic cancer, has a personal history of major depression in his 20s, and is a daily user of alcohol with around five to six standard drinks per day. He is now having low mood, anergia, weight loss, lack of interest in spending time with friends/family, and he missed a recent appointment for lab work in order to start treatment. Here, the differential includes recurrent major depressive disorder, adjustment disorder, and substance-induced mood disorder (alcohol). Given the high symptom burden, immediate intervention with a multimodal approach including counseling around alcohol use, coping support, and psychotropic medications will be most likely to improve function and prevent further decline, despite diagnostic uncertainty. As with mhGAP implementation, addressing mental health needs in seriously ill patients in the primary care setting using a palliative care approach requires adaptation.

The Collaborative Care Model (CoCM)[8] is another important concept when considering mental health and primary palliative care. CoCM offers a strategy to expand mental health care delivery within the existing primary care systems using four core features: team-based, evidence-based, measurement-driven, and population-level.[9] CoCM workforce is structured with a core team consisting of the primary care providers (PCPs), the care manager (CM), and the psychiatrist. Where traditional thinking, often described as 'the iron triangle', dictates that only two out of three priorities of care – cost, access, and quality[10] – can be optimized at the same time, the CoCM seeks to optimize all three. CoCM minimizes costs by leveraging the limited psychiatrist time, expands access by having the whole primary care team evaluate and treat patients, and maintains quality by utilizing the psychiatrist's expertise to ensure evidence-based care. This same CoCM can be adapted for palliative care, especially in oncology and ICU settings.

PALLIATIVE CARE IN THE COVID ERA

Primary care plays a vital role in palliative care services, although it is not always a key issue in all healthcare settings. It is undisputed that the palliative care approach has been negatively influenced by the COVID-19 pandemic, particularly focusing on healthcare professionals. A study by Sena and De Luca[11] aimed to explore the perceptions of palliative care health professionals and physicians regarding end-of-life care management in COVID units during the first two waves of the pandemic in Italy. They suggested that the COVID-19 crisis highlighted the need to deepen and, possibly, redefine the professional, ethical, and clinical roles of palliative care teams, not only in managing COVID patients but also in the healthcare system as a whole.

In line with the notion that palliative care entered a phase of change during the COVID-19 era, a systematic review by Perdikouri et al.[12] examined the impact on palliative care services from the healthcare professionals' perspective. The authors emphasized that 'despite the important role palliative care can play during a health crisis, it was not always adequately reflected in pandemic plans'. According to this study, the effects of increased workload, altered delivery of care, and implications for the mental health of the staff involved require prompt attention and should be considered in future pandemic planning.

Moreover, Mitchell and Barclay[13] argue that the COVID-19 pandemic presents an opportunity for those who provide palliative care to rethink how to move beyond the traditional service model. They advocate for more efforts to integrate with primary care teams and networks and call for robust engagement in multidisciplinary research. They state, 'new primary care, community, and specialist palliative care partnerships are needed to deliver novel, integrated services that make optimal use of the limited workforce to provide patient care'.

Another significant issue is the impact of the COVID-19 pandemic on the provision of compassionate care and the burnout of healthcare professionals, especially those involved in palliative care and end-of-life services. A literature review by Lluch et al.[14] aimed to assess burnout, compassion fatigue, and compassion satisfaction levels, as well as their associated risks and protective factors, in healthcare professionals during the first year of the COVID-19 pandemic. They reported increased burnout rates, dimensions of emotional exhaustion, depersonalization, and compassion fatigue, a reduction in personal accomplishment, and levels of compassion satisfaction similar to pre-pandemic times. The main risk factors associated with burnout were anxiety, depression, and insomnia, along with sociodemographic variables such as being female, a nurse, or working directly with COVID-19 patients. Similar results were found for compassion fatigue. The study found that the main protective factors were resilience and social support.

In a cross-sectional study by Arnal et al.,[15] the impact of the COVID-19 pandemic on the Spanish palliative care professionals' capacity to perform compassionate care and their well-being was explored. Compassion was predicted by the ability to control the workload and cope with death, while burnout was predicted by age, workload, control over workload, self-care, material resources, and changes in teamwork. According to this study, factors like age, workload control, changes in teamwork, and self-care were significant predictors of compassion satisfaction. Different variables were shown to predict compassion fatigue: compassion, control over workload, social self-care, and the ability to cope with death. Both above studies highlight the importance of focusing on the impact of the COVID-19 pandemic on compassion satisfaction and fatigue, as well as burnout –key issues when discussing palliative care and end of life in a period of crisis.

In spite of great efforts from different health systems to develop new possibilities of communications with patients to avoid the effects of lockdown, including telemedicine, it seems that these tools have had limited success. Perception from both sides, patients and professionals, of a lack of proximity made them not feel comfortable in dealing with tele-consultations.[16,17] This was particularly frequently experienced in primary care and mainly when dealing with patients in difficult situations including end-of-life moments and need of palliative care.

Higginson and colleagues highlighted the lack of systematic evidence to understand the quality of end-of-life care delivery during COVID-19 pandemics.[18] Although role of primary care in end-of-life care is crucial, it has received little attention in policy during the COVID or during previous pandemic situations.[19] As Mitchel and colleagues also indicated, 'frontline primary care has the potential to deliver high quality community end-of-life care for all who need it'.[20] To active such a desirable outcome, there is a need for adequate allocation of sources including funding and professional workforce in primary care settings.

REFERENCES

1. WHO publication. Available at: https://www.who.int/publications/i/item/integrating-palliative-care-and-symptom-relief-into-primary-health-care
2. Slort W, Schweitzer B, Blankenstein A, et al. Perceived barriers and facilitators for general practitioner–patient communication in palliative care: a systematic review. Palliat Med. 2011;25(6):613–629.
3. https://pinkbook.dfci.org
4. https://www.mypcnow.org/fast-facts/
5. Childers JW, Back AL, Tulsky JA, Arnold RM. REMAP: a framework for goals of care conversations. J Oncol Pract. 2017 Oct;13(10):e844–e850. doi: 10.1200/JOP.2016.018796
6. Paladino J, Fromme EK. Preparing for serious illness: a model for better conversations over the continuum of care. Am Fam Physician. 2019 Mar 1. www.aafp.org/pubs/afp/issues/2019/0301/p281.html
7. Dalgleish T, Black M, Johnston D, Bevan A. Transdiagnostic approaches to mental health problems: current status and future directions. J Consult Clin Psychol. 2020 Mar;88(3):179–195. doi: 10.1037/ccp0000482
8. Raney L. Integrating primary care and behavioral health: the role of psychiatrists in the collaborative care model. Am J Psych. 2015;172(8):721–728.
9. Acharya B, Ekstrand M, Rimal P, et al. Collaborative care for mental health in low- and middle-income countries: a WHO Health Systems Framework assessment of three programs. Psychiatr Serv. 2017;68:870–872.
10. van der Goes DN, Edwardson N, Rayamajhee V, Hollis C, Hunter D. An iron triangle ROI model for health care. Clinicoecon Outcomes Res. 2019;11:335–348.
11. Sena B, De Luca E. Managing the end of life in COVID patients. The role of palliative care in emergency departments during the pandemic. Front Sociol. 2022 Nov 9;7:1039003.
12. Perdikouri K, et al. The impact of COVID-19 pandemic on palliative care services as perceived by healthcare professionals: a systematic review. Int J Caring Sci. 2023;16(1):121–138.
13. Mitchell S, Barclay S, Evans C, Sleeman K. Palliative and end-of-life care in primary care during the COVID-19 pandemic and beyond. Br J Gen Pract. 2021 Dec 31;72(714):6–7.
14. Lluch C, Galiana L, Doménech P, Sansó N. The impact of the COVID-19 pandemic on Burnout, compassion fatigue, and compassion satisfaction in healthcare personnel: a systematic review of the literature published during the first year of the pandemic. Healthcare (Basel). 2022 Feb 13;10(2):364.
15. Campos I Arnal A, Galiana L, Sánchez-Ruiz J, Sansó N. Cross-sectional study of the professional quality of life of palliative care professionals during the COVID-19 pandemic. Healthcare (Basel). 2023 Dec 19;12(1):4.
16. Garattini L, Badinella Martini M, Zanetti M. More room for telemedicine after COVID-19: lessons for primary care. Eur J Health Econ. 2021 Mar;22(2):183–186. doi: 10.1007/s10198-020-01248-y
17. Vosburg RW, Robinson KA. Telemedicine in primary care during the COVID-19 pandemic: provider and patient satisfaction examined. Telemed J E Health. 2022 Feb;28(2):167–175.
18. Higginson IJ, Brooks D, Barclay S. Dying at home during the pandemic. BMJ. 2021;373:n1437.

19. Mitchell S, Maynard V, Lyons V, et al. The role and response of primary healthcare services in the delivery of palliative care in epidemics and pandemics: a rapid review to inform practice and service delivery during the COVID-19 pandemic. Palliat Med. 2020;34–9:1182–1192.
20. Mitchell S, Chapman H, Fowler I, McTague L. Dying at home during COVID-19: a view from primary care. BMJ. 2021 Jul 14;374:n1776.

CHAPTER 9

Thanatophobia

Exacerbation/amplification of existing anxiety disorders/phobias with a focus on GPs' key role in encouraging patients to seek help and adhere to healthy behaviours

Abdullah Dukhail AlKhathami, Christos Lionis, and Ana B. Pérez Villalva

INTRODUCTION

Sara, a married woman with two adolescent children, seeks help for persistent feelings of dread and intrusive thoughts about death. Her anxiety has escalated over the past year following the sudden death of a close friend in a car accident. She reports difficulty sleeping, recurring nightmares of her own death, and avoidance of activities she previously enjoyed, such as driving and socializing. As a high-achieving marketing executive, Sara has begun to struggle professionally due to intrusive thoughts and lack of concentration. Her family describe her as increasingly withdrawn and irritable.

Thanatophobia, death anxiety, is an expression of people's fear of death. Either they worry about dying for themselves, or they worry about losing people they love, in a disturbing way that negatively affects their life. The fear of death and the anxiety that follows it is common from time to time, and beliefs and practices concerning death have changed throughout human history.[1] It is natural for a person to strive for survival despite the certainty that their life will end one day.[2] Research has shown that 10% of people suffer from death anxiety, and about 3% have an intense fear of death.[3]

DOI: 10.1201/9781003473947-13

Death anxiety can be an isolated problem or a part of other mental health disorders such as depression, panic, and general anxiety disorder.[4] It constitutes a problem that requires intervention and treatment if it has a clear impact, takes a long time, or hinders required life obligations.[1] The fear associated with dying and the anxiety with which it is related are characteristic features of the attitude toward death.[5] As has been seen throughout history, human beings have reflected on the meaning of mortality. They have developed elaborate defense mechanisms against the terror of death at the individual and social levels.

The problem with death denial is that no matter how hard we try to suppress and repress awareness of death, anxiety about our death can still manifest itself in a variety of symptoms, bringing with it significant behavioural and emotional consequences.[5,6] Sooner or later, events in life, such as a terminal illness or the death of a loved one, push us right in the face of the harsh reality of mortality.

Death is a sensitive subject due to its universal scope.[7] Dying is part of the natural processes that accompany life. It is an individualized psychological and physical experience that reflects social and cultural identity. At the same time, it is a stressful situation that poses the greatest threat and challenge for humanity since it affects both the person who is dying and the people who care for them.[8,9]

HISTORICAL PERSPECTIVES

Table 9.1 presents a chronological overview of significant milestones in the historical development of scholarly interest in death anxiety. The timeline spans from the early psychoanalytic reflections of Sigmund Freud in 1918 through to the evolving concepts of a "good death" in the late 20th century. This historical progression reflects a gradual shift from philosophical and psychoanalytic contemplation of mortality to a more empirical and socio-culturally nuanced understanding of death-related attitudes and practices.

The table illustrates how death, initially conceptualized as a repressed or taboo subject within Western societies, gradually became the focus of critical inquiry across disciplines such as history, anthropology, sociology, and psychology. Pioneers like Philippe Ariès, Herman Feifel, and Elisabeth Kübler-Ross played pivotal roles in highlighting the denial and medicalization of death, while later scholars expanded the discourse to include cultural diversity, palliative care, and the pursuit of dignity at the end of life.

This historical lens not only underscores the evolving academic and societal narratives surrounding death but also provides essential context for understanding contemporary approaches to death anxiety, palliative care, and death education. The table serves as a foundation for exploring how death has been interpreted, avoided, or ritualized in various cultural and temporal contexts.

TABLE 9.1 History of the studies of death anxiety

Year	Event
1918	Freud reflects on death and on the First World War. Formulates the denial of death for the first time in psychoanalysis, affirming that deep down no one believes in their own death. In the unconscious they are convinced of immortality. It is religious and philosophical beliefs that aim to avoid the prospect of death due to the inability to accept and understand death.
1919	This topic is introduced with the book The Waning of the Middle Ages, written by the Dutch historian Johan Huizinga. His work explored the visions of death held in France and the Netherlands in past centuries. It was marked by plagues, war, and some legends surrounding death (forging the macabre for posterity). Thus, more works continued to be written with a macabre style-associated with death. It continued to be an attractive field of research for historians of 'mentalities' (a term named after the French Academy, it can also be understood as attitudes) for sociologists and anthropologists.
1949	The French historian Philippe Ariès published a book on attitudes toward death.
1955	The British anthropologist Geoffrey Gores describes death as the new taboo of Western society.
1958	William A. Faunce and Robert L. Fulton highlighted how less exposure to the process of death and dying was maintained (e.g., in the West the care of the deceased is carried out through funeral homes, replacing the family in funeral rituals). On the other hand, the use of euphemisms describing the death of someone, embalming to preserve life, and the dissolution of traditional customs made Western mourning characterized by 'conflict, frustration, and anxiety'.
1959	Herman Feifel, in his book Concern for Death, wrote that death had been relegated to the territory of taboos, so people kept their thoughts, fears, and emotions about it to themselves. Charles Wahl reinforces the same idea stating how harmful the taboo is on an emotional level. Since it consumes the task of living in a free, creative, and unhindered way.
1960s	The denial of death was reinforced due to the spread of a critical movement related to medicalized death. The term good death, emerged in the United States and Europe as a key concept of the nascent hospice and palliative movement.[9]
1967	Philippe Ariès mentioned that there was a strong cultural denial of death in the United States. Both Gorier and Ariès elaborated on the notion of a contemporary denial of death and its consequences, which would remain hegemonic in death studies at least until the 1990s.
1969	Elisabeth Kübler-Ross published her essay On Death and the Dying, which drives the palliative care movement, giving rise to the interview protocol with terminal patients, carried out in 1965. The attitudes she found coincided with those of Ariès.

(Continued)

TABLE 9.1 History of the studies of death anxiety *(Continued)*

Year	Event
1975	In France, the anthropologist Louis-Vincent Thomas and the sociologist Jean Ziegler mentioned the deleterious repression effects of death in Western capitalist societies, in contrast with the ritualized death present in African peoples or the indigenous nations of Brazil.
1983	O'Neil made the first approach to the concept that death was good if the individual maintained control and autonomy over the dying process and the moment of death. He was referring to euthanasia.
	Later, Kellehear suggests that a good death in hospitals can be achieved under the following conditions: awareness of dying, preparation for death, abandonment of roles and responsibilities, and dismissal. Although there is no clear definition, similar expressions are used in the literature, such as die well, die in peace, appropriate death, desired death, or dignified death. The concept of a good death presents some variations among subgroups, given their ethnic, cultural, and socioeconomic characteristics. Thus, the multicultural nature of many societies shapes the experience of dying in complex ways.[9]
2004	Camilla Zimmermann and Gary Rodin found that conversations about death and the end of life were often intended to be avoided or silenced. Making a conspiracy of silence surrounding these issues and that death was not discussed in public.
2007	Zimmermann perceives some harmful aspects (such as not wanting to talk about one's mortality), which delimits the narrative through morality, defining a correct or incorrect way of dying.[11]

Source: Adapted from Cozzolino et al.[10]

ANXIETY PATHOPHYSIOLOGY

Anxiety disorders are the most common mental health disorder, the main features of which include excessive fear and worry or avoidance of threats,[11] including death. Anxiety disorders are often comorbid with other mental disorders, especially depression, as well as with physical disorders, which generally worsen the severity of the symptoms, clinical burden, and management outcomes.[12,13]

Neuroimaging techniques have greatly contributed to the knowledge and understanding of the neural circuits of anxiety-related disorders. They indicate significant changes in the function and structure of the limbic structures of people with fear and anxiety,[14] with increased right amygdala activation correlated with the severity of anxiety reflected in masked angry faces.[15] Neuroimaging has also shown that the amygdala and its connections have an important role in emotional, associative, attentional, and interpretive processes.[16] When a defect occurs in this circuit, one of its consequences is anxiety disorders, resulting in impaired communication with the frontal areas responsible for inhibitory responses, and an increased response of the amygdala, which results in a continuous process of processing related to the threat.[17] Therefore, the amygdala has a role in acquiring and expressing conditioned fear.[18]

Norepinephrine, serotonin, dopamine, and gamma-aminobutyric acid (GABA) are major mediators of anxiety symptoms through the autonomic nervous system, particularly the sympathetic nervous system; corticotropin-releasing factor may be also involved.[17,19]

DIAGNOSTIC CRITERIA

Death anxiety often begins in childhood with factors affecting the establishment and development of this fear such as genetics, early childhood experiences, traumatic events, and culture and religious beliefs.

Menzies and Veale[1] identify eight mental processes, any one of which indicates the presence of thanatophobia:

- Thinking a lot about death on a daily basis.
- Images in mind about ways of dying or of after death.
- Avoiding things thought to cause death.
- Avoiding anything reminiscent of death.
- Excessively seeking reassurance that someone is safe, healthy, and loved.
- Doing things that will maintain health and safety in an excessive way.
- Searching more information on death or after death.
- Acting in ways to try to improve the outcome after death.

ATTITUDES TOWARD DEATH

How we relate to our mortality is mediated by the same factors, adding that the circumstances surrounding the death of a loved one could also have had an influence.[6,20] Attitudes toward death are varied. A person shapes their attitude toward death depending on what elements of their attitude they perceives and how they experience them. The complexity of death's phenomenon and the singularity of the human person conditioned the attitudes. To die defines personal meaning and determines how we live.[8,9] Thinking about death allows us to be aware of the reality of mortality.[21] Indisputably, attitudes toward death are linked to its cause. Some diseases, such as those of sexual transmission, still maintain a social stigma in patients and their families.[21] Other diseases cause social empathy, as those who die from an oncological condition or a chronic degenerative disease.

Added to the above, it has been seen that in developed countries having a 'good death' maintains a relationship with the process of dying (in itself) and can minimize any sense of struggle.[22] Although what constitutes a good death for each person is an individual experience, which can change over time (even once a person knows that they are going to die, their decisions and perspectives can change in a prolonged dying process), without losing sight of the fact that it is based on perspectives, cultural contexts, and experiences acquired in the course of their life histories, the latter can contribute to the development of death anxiety.[8,23]

Taking the existential approach, Wong and his team[24] defined and studied different attitudes toward death:

- Neutral acceptance of death which implies rationally accepting death as a natural, integral, and immutable part of life. Generating an indifferent attitude toward death.[21]
- Approaching acceptance, the death is accepted as a gateway to a better life after death.[6]
- Escape from acceptance since death is chosen as a better alternative to a painful existence.[6]

THANATOPHOBIA INTERVENTIONS IN PRIMARY CARE

Fear of death is one of the issues that needs collaborative treatment between the family doctor and a psychologist. Firstly, associated mental disorders such as general anxiety, depression, panic attacks, and others are treated. Then cooperation with the psychologist in self-support and acceptance of the idea of death in a positive way.[25]

Terror Management Theory (TMT) states that people have a certain level of awareness of their impending mortality.[26] Individuals become defensive and predominantly seek meaning in symbolic sources extrinsic to the self. Also, there are aspects of people's experiences that remind them of their mortality, and this creates anxiety. For example, the simple act of passing a funeral home can create a reminder of one's mortality. Avoiding death anxiety is the primary motive, while the search for positive meaning is the secondary motive because the latter is used to protect ourselves from the terror of death.[27,28] Consequently, people seek to reduce anxiety related to their mortality by becoming attached to or investing in something that will outlast their short existence (e.g., a cultural worldview), to cope with the terror associated with their mortality.

There are variety of evidence-based therapeutic interventions including existential psychotherapy and cognitive-behavioural therapy.[29] It is important to recalibrate oneself with new self-esteem to gain a greater sense of self through self-concept, clarity of self-concept, locus of control (especially intrinsic), self-actualization, and existential well-being.[28] Those with a more internal locus of control and higher intrinsic religiosity have lower levels of anxiety about known and unknown death.[29]

SARA

We now return to the case of Sara.

Clinical Observations and Assessment

- *Psychological Symptoms*: Generalized anxiety, avoidance behaviours, intrusive thoughts about death, and hypervigilance.
- *Physical Symptoms*: Insomnia, somatic complaints, and fatigue.

Contributing Factors

- *Cognitive and Emotional Factors*: Catastrophic thinking about death and perfectionistic tendencies fuel her inability to tolerate uncertainty about the future
- *Sociocultural Influences*: The culture in combination with limited emotional openness in her family contribute to the internalization of her fears.
- *Life Events*: The unexpected death of her close friend acted as a triggering event.

Applying the Al-Khathami 5-Step approach[30] to Sara's case

- *Anticipating the Need for Psychological Care*: A psychological issue could be suspected based on her psychological symptoms, the recent trauma of her close friend, frequent visits to the clinic for somatic complaints without any identifiable physical cause.
- *Screening for Psychological Stress*: A focused screening during the interview to explore Sara's hidden complaints and delusions about death.
- *Scoping*: Referral or primary care management.
- *Diagnosis*: The doctor identifies:
  - Primary Diagnosis: Death anxiety (thanatophobia).
  - Comorbid Diagnosis: Mild to moderate depression, exacerbated by the grief of her friend's death and unaddressed existential concerns.
  - No psychosis, self-harm behaviours, or severe depression requiring immediate psychiatric referral are present.
- *Management*: The doctor decides that Sara can be managed at the primary care level with appropriate interventions, while keeping an option for mental health specialist referral if necessary.

In the initial phase:

- *Building Rapport and Psychoeducation*: Focused on establishing a safe therapeutic environment and educating Sara about the nature of death anxiety. Normalizing her fears and introducing the concept of death as a universal concern were key strategies.

- *Cognitive-Behavioural Therapy (CBT)*: CBT techniques addressed Sara's cognitive distortions, such as catastrophic thinking about death.
- *Existential Therapy*: Existential discussions to explore Sara's beliefs about life, purpose, and death. She was encouraged to reflect on her values.
- *Mindfulness and Relaxation Techniques*: These helped Sara stay present and reduce her anxiety about the uncontrollable aspects of the future.
- *Family Support and Communication*: Through family sessions they improved their communication, received education about death anxiety and guidance on how to meet Sara's emotional needs.

- *Follow-Up Plan*: Scheduling bi-weekly follow-ups to assess Sara's progress, refine strategies, and determine if referral to a specialist becomes necessary. Monitoring for signs of improvement.
- *Outcome*: After six months of therapy, Sara reports a significant reduction in intrusive thoughts and anxiety levels. She resumes her activities and accepts mortality as a natural part of life. While occasional fears persist, Sara demonstrates improved coping skills.

CONCLUSION

Death anxiety is a complex phenomenon that requires a holistic therapeutic approach. Sara's case underscores the significance of integrating cognitive-behavioural and existential techniques to foster psychological resilience and acceptance in individuals facing this pervasive fear.

Death exposes the fragility of life and the uselessness of daily occupations and efforts. Death focuses and clarifies. People with a positive orientation are willing to face the crisis and create growth opportunities. They are primarily motivated by their desire to fulfil their life mission, a meaningful life, regardless of the risks, because they have found something worth dying for. The positive orientation is more focused on what makes life worth living despite the suffering and anxiety of death.[6]

REFERENCES

1. Menzies RE, Veale D. Free yourself from death anxiety: a CBT Self-Help Guide for a fear of death and Dying. London, Jessica Kingsley Publishers, 2022.
2. White J. A practical guide to death and dying. Coral Gables, Quest. 1980.
3. Noyes Jr R, Hartz AJ, Doebbeling CC, Malis RW, Happel RL, Werner LA, Yagla SJ. Illness fears in the general population. Psychosom Med. 2000; 62, 318–325.
4. Iverach L, Menzies RG, Menzies RE. Death anxiety and its role in psychopathology: reviewing the status of a transdiagnostic construct. Clin Psychol Rev. 2014; 34, 580–593.
5. Robert M, Tradii L. Do we deny death? I. A genealogy of death denial, Mortality. 2017; 24, 1–14.

6. Sawyer JS, Brewster ME, Ertl MM. Death anxiety and death acceptance in atheists and other nonbelievers. Death Stud. 2021; 45(6), 459–468.

7. Rainsford S, MacLeod RD, Glasgow NJ, Wilson DM, Phillips CB, Wiles RB. Rural residents' perspectives on the rural 'good death': a scoping review. Health & Social Care in the Community. 2018; 26(3), 273–294.

8. Schott G. I know death. He's got many faces:' The presence of death in young peoples' media. Mortality. 2021; 26(4), 367–375.

9. Tradii L, Robert M. Do we deny death? II. Critiques of the death-denial thesis. Mortality. 2017; 24, 277–388.

10. Cozzolino PJ, Blackie LER, Meyers LS. Self-related consequences of death fear and death denial. Death Stud. 2014; 38(6), 418–422.

11. Kessler RC, Demler O, Frank RG, et al. Prevalence and treatment of mental disorders, 1990 to 2003. N Engl J Med. 2005; 352, 2515–2523.

12. Penninx B, Pine D, Holmes E, Reif A. Anxiety disorders. Lancet. 2021; 397(10277), 914–927.

13. Grillon C. Startle reactivity and anxiety disorders: aversive conditioning, context, and neurobiology. Biol Psychiatry. 2002; 52(10), 958–975.

14. Freitas-Ferrari MC, Hallak JE, Trzesniak C, Filho AS, Machado-de-Sousa JP, et al. Neuroimaging in social anxiety disorder: a systematic review of the literature. Progress Neuro-Psychopharm Biol Psychiatry. 2010; 34, 565–580.

15. Monk CS, Telzer EH, Mogg K, Bradley BP, Mai X, Louro HM, et al. Amygdala and ventrolateral prefrontal cortex activation to masked angry faces in children and adolescents with generalized anxiety disorder. Arch Gen Psychiatry. 2008; 65, 568–576.

16. de Carvalho MR, Rozenthal M, Nardi AE. The fear circuitry in panic disorder and its modulation by cognitive-behaviour therapy interventions. World J Biol Psychiatry. 2010; 11(2 Pt 2), 188–198.

17. Akirav I, Maroun M. The role of the medial prefrontal cortex-amygdala circuit in stress effects on the extinction of fear. Neural Plast. 2007; 2007, 30873.

18. Cammarota M, Bevilaqua LR, Vianna MR, Medina JH, Izquierdo I. The extinction of conditioned fear: structural and molecular basis and therapeutic use. Rev Bras Psiquiatr. 2007; 29(1), 80–85.

19. Michael T, Zetsche U, Margraf J. Epidemiology of anxiety disorders. Psychiatry Epidemiology and psychopharmacology. 2007; 7(4), 136–142.

20. Jong J, Ross R, Philip T, Chang S-H, Simons N, Halberstadt J. The religious correlates of death anxiety: a systematic review and meta-analysis. Relig Brain Behav. 2018; 8, 4–20.

21. Jong J. Death anxiety and religion. Current opinion in Psychology. 2021; 40, 40–44.

22. McTeague L, Lang P, Wangelin B, Laplante M, Bradley M. Defensive mobilization in specific phobia: fear specificity, negative affectivity, and diagnostic prominence. Biol Psychiatry. 2012; 72(1), 8–18.

23. Sušnik M. Death as a fact of life: a perspective on the badness of death, Mortality. 2020; 27(3), 322–335.

24. Wong PTP. Existential positive psychology and integrative meaning therapy. Int Rev Psychiatry. 2020; 32(7-8), 565–578.

25. Archer C, Kessler D, Wiles N & Turner K. GPs' and patients' views on the value of diagnosing anxiety disorders in primary care: a qualitative interview study. Br J Gen Practice. 2021; 71(707), 450–457.

26. Pyszczynski T, Greenberg J, Solomon S, Maxfield M. On the unique psychological import of the human awareness of mortality: themes and variations. Psychol Inquiry. 2006; 17, 328–356.

27. Ikwuemesi CK. Celebrating tragedy: dying, death and mortuary arts among the Igbo, Mortality. 2021; 28, 1–28.

28. Benton JP, Christopher AN, Walter MI. Death anxiety as a function of aging anxiety. Death Stud. 2007; 31(4), 337–350.

29. Menzies RE, Zuccala M, Sharpe L, Dar-Nimrod I. The effects of psychosocial interventions on death anxiety: A meta-analysis and systematic review of randomised controlled trials. J Anxiety Disorders. 2018; 59, 64–73.

30. Al-Khathami AD. An innovative 5-Step Patient Interview approach for integrating mental healthcare into primary care centre services: a validation study. Gen Psychiatry. 2022; 35, e100693.

CHAPTER 10

Child mental health

Flávio Dias Silva, Laura Canessa, Deepika Shaligram, and Ana B. Pérez Villalva

INTRODUCTION

Paulo was a cheerful 9-year-old boy who did well at school, enjoyed football and even aroused enthusiasm in his local community, who saw in him a promising future as an athlete. However, his country went to war and his town was severely affected, leading Paulo to immigrate with his family to another country with a different language and customs. His father had to stay in his home country to look after his grandparents. Paulo's mother brings him to an appointment with the family doctor in the new country, complaining that Paulo has been losing weight because he eats too little. He has also been crying at home, isolating himself from his family and even refusing to go to school on some days.

Childhood is a critical period for physical and mental development. Good mental health is foundational for overall health and well-being across the lifespan. The prevalence of pediatric mental health disorders is almost 15% globally [1, 2]. Although 50% of mental health disorders begin by the age of 14 and 75% by the age of 24 [2], there is limited access to mental health treatment due to healthcare workforce shortages around the world. Thus, youth mental health has been declared a global priority with a particular urgency precipitated by the COVID-19 pandemic. To meet the post-pandemic needs, the field of child and adolescent mental health services is expected to grow in the domains of population-based care, integration of virtual, digital application-based psychotherapies and short-term interventions, and disaster psychiatry, with a special emphasis on collaboration with primary care [3].

MENTAL HEALTH CARE OF CHILDREN AND ADOLESCENTS – OPPORTUNITIES OF APPROACH IN PRIMARY CARE

Patients present to their primary care providers more frequently with recent symptoms and signs than with long-term established or diagnosed disorders. Considering this, the first task for family doctors is to perform the initial evaluation of the youth/family complaints. A 'presenting problem approach' seems the most suitable model in this context. Table 10.1 shows some of the most common chief complaints of child/adolescent mental health issues by age.

TABLE 10.1 Selected mental health reasons for seeking primary care

Infant (0–2 years old)	Early childhood (2–5 years old)	Young child (6–12) years old)	Adolescent (13–18 years old)
• Delayed milestones • Insomnia • Irritability • Feed refusal	• Irritability • Aggressiveness • Delayed milestones (especially speech delay) • Fears	• Impaired concentration • Aggressiveness • School refusal • Insomnia • Fears • Medically unexplained symptoms	• Irritability • Sadness • Insomnia • Self-harm • Social withdrawal • Impaired concentration • School refusal • Eating problems

Source: Compiled by the authors, with references of Kramer and Garralda [4].

Once the problem(s) is/are well defined, a thorough evaluation is the next step. Often mental or behavioural issues in children may be normal and healthy reactions to life events, such as a time- and intensity-limited fear of dogs. On other hand, when behavioural problems are more severe than expected, the clinician must be aware of possible emerging disorders. To understand the impact of the symptoms in a child/adolescent's life is crucial to an appropriate approach. A helpful framework to focus on this point is 'Patient Centered Medicine' (PCM), a method that is already used by many family doctors [5]. In PCM, doctors follow four steps to develop clinical reasoning and management: (1) exploring the patient's experience of illness, (2) understanding the patient as a whole person, (3) building a joint care plan with the patient, and (4) fostering a strong patient–provider relationship. In the next two sections, a proposal is presented using this method to approach mental health care for young people in primary care.

Diagnostic approaches – defining the presenting problem, its impact, and probable nature

The *first component* of PCM is understanding the illness and how the patient is being affected by it. This will allow the doctor to comprise the latent reason for consultation. Sometimes patients and families visit doctors only wanting to know if there is a major problem; in other instances, they really may want help to deal with a specific issue; and finally, sometimes they are referred by someone, like the school or juvenile justice system, and may be not aware of the reason for consultation. Understanding the needs of the patient and their family is essential for the effectiveness of the approach. This can be accomplished by assessing the impairments caused by the related symptoms in daily life, relationships, and/or personal health, as academic underachievement, for example. Keeping key child/adolescent developmental milestones in mind can help in considering differential diagnosis. Table 10.2 lists some important age-specific milestones to be considered in diagnostic evaluation.

Assessment tools (like structured questionnaires to patients, caregivers or even teachers) can help to evaluate symptoms better and grade their severity. Symptom characteristics can also point to the need for additional laboratory tests and neuroimaging, to rule out differential diagnosis. Table 10.3 provides a list of potentially useful validated evaluation instruments, some of which are translated into many languages. It is important to remember that these tools provide clinically useful information, but they are not diagnostic *per se*.

The *second component* of PCM indeed states that the clinician must know the patient as a whole – personality, family, and community. Given the importance of these variables on a child's mental development, remembering concepts of these three great influences is essential for providing good care:

• *Personality* is the combination of characteristics or qualities that form an individual's distinctive character. It is influenced by temperament – the innate pattern of human behavior – and life experiences, especially the early childhood ones. Genetics and perinatal conditions can predispose to temperament styles and neurodevelopmental disorders such as autism. On other hand, adverse experiences such as trauma or neglect can predispose to future emotional problems like depression or even personality disorders. Considering the temperament and personal history of a child – who the child is – is very important to understand the presenting problems and for treatment planning.

TABLE 10.2 Age-specific milestones to be considered in diagnostic evaluation

		Language/Cognition	Social-Emotional
Infant (0–2 years old)	4 months	Begins to recognize their own body and to develop eye-hand-eye and audio-visual coordination. Responds to stimuli by cooing.	The first interaction behaviors appear, interest in sound, vowel games.
	6 months	Imitates gestures and sounds of adults and perceives that objects remain even when they are momentarily out of their sight (object permanence).	Recognizes family members, observes or smiles in front of a mirror.
	12 months	Makes sounds, repeats words, and gestures what they want. Walks without help, drinks from the cup. Responds to 'no'.	Begins the process of socialization and individuation. Imitates gestures.
	18 months	Follows simple commands. Improves balance and coordination for motor activities and acquires more complex skills.	Stage of incorporation into the family, the development of their identity begins. Important: To prioritize the daily routines of care and interaction.
Early childhood (2–5 years old)	2 years old	Egocentric thinking: static, intuitive and lacking in logic. Symbolic function appears through deferred imitation (mental image), play, drawing, language. Attribute human feelings or thoughts to objects.	Developing their identity and independence, acquiring a place within the family. Enjoys collaborating with adults in simple tasks. Plays in parallel.
	3 years old	Accelerated development of language: relates experiences, desires, and past experiences.	Sociable, talkative, begins to become aware of others. Attempts to control emotions.

4 years old	Very good motor balance, interested in letters and numbers. Asks, 'Why?' Still cannot adequately differentiate reality from fantasy.	Listens to others and is able to share games.
5 years old	Begins to be interested in new learning (learning to read and write).	Develops independence and perfects autonomy. Has initiative, needs parental approval. Important: To promote the development of symbolic function, creativity, and growing autonomy.
Young child (6–12 years old)	Is able to reason and follow rules and regulations. Can see things from the other person's perspective. Thinking with greater flexibility. Begin to use limited logical thought processes and can sort, group, and classify based on common characteristics.	They can control themselves, and begin to develop a sense of morals and a code of values. They adapt more to cultural norms, rules, and laws, and become increasingly interested in social activities with their peers. Important: Period of great changes and behavioural reorganizations, and a growing interest in peer relationships.
Adolescent (13–18 years old)	Accelerated rate of growth and changes that began with puberty: bodily, hormonal, cognitive, and sexual. Hypothetical deductive thinking.	Adolescent tasks: Search for self-identity Separation from attachment figures Path to independence Reorganization of sexual drives. Important: Stage that pursues the definitive entry into the social world.

Source: Compiled by the authors, with references to Shaffer and Kipp [6].

TABLE 10.3 Selected instruments for evaluating child/adolescent mental health complaints

Instrument	Scope	Resource
Strengths and Difficulties Questionnaire (SDQ) Goodman, 1997	Evaluates prosocial behavior and problems in emotions, peer relationships, hyperactivity, and conduct.	www.sdqinfo.com
Mood and Feelings Questionnaire Angold et al., 1995	A measure assessing recent depressive symptomatology in children aged 6–17 years with self and parent versions.	https://psychiatry.duke.edu/research/research-programs-areas/assessment-intervention/developmental-epidemiology-instruments-0
Screen for Child Anxiety-Related Emotion Disorders (SCARED) Birmaher et al., 1997	Children and parent versions assess anxiety disorders including general anxiety disorder, separation anxiety disorder, panic disorder, and social phobia, besides specific school phobia.	https://www.aacap.org/App_Themes/AACAP/docs/member_resources/toolbox_for_clinical_practice_and_outcomes/symptoms/ScaredChild.pdf
Swanson, Nolan, and Pelham–IV Questionnaire (SNAP IV) Swanson, 1992	The longer version allows a better general view of a child's behavior. The 26-item scale focuses on attention-deficit/hyperactivity disorder (ADHD) and oppositional defiant disorder (ODD).	http://www.caddra.ca/pdfs/caddraGuidelines2011SNAP.pdf
Child Stress Disorders Checklist Short Form (CSDC-SF) Bosquet, Kassam-Adams, & Saxe, 2010	SF comes from the original 36-item CSDC but maintains its power to detect stress-/trauma-related disorders.	https://www.healthcaretoolbox.org/images/pdf/CSDC_SF.pdf
Children's Revised Impact of Event Scale (CRIES-8) Yule et al., 1997	Based on *Impact of Event Scale*, CRIES-8 evaluates risk for trauma- or stress-related disorder.	http://www.childrenandwar.org/measures/children%E2%80%99s-revised-impact-of-event-scale-8-%E2%80%93-cries-8/

CRAFFT Test Knight et al, 2002	Acronyms of six points (Car, Relax, Alone, Forget, Friends, Trouble) to evaluate alcohol or drugs misuse.	http://www.ceasar-boston.org/CRAFFT/index.php
Modified Checklist for Autism in Toddlers, Revised with Follow-Up (M-CHAT-R/F) Robins et al., 2013	Reduces the false-positive rate and detects more autism spectrum disorders (ASD) cases than the original tool.	http://mchatscreen.com/
Childhood Autism Spectrum Test (CAST) Willians et al., 2005	Developed by University of Cambridge Autism Research Centre among several other tests for ASD detection.	https://www.autismresearchcentre.com/arc_tests
Eating Attitudes Test (EAT)/Child Eating Attitudes Test (ChEAT) Garner & Garfinkel, 1982 / Maloney et al., 1988	Easy-to-use screening tool in primary care or schools.	http://www.eat-26.com/ and https://novopsych.com/assessments/child/children-eating-attitudes-test-cheat/

Source: Compiled by the authors, with references of Guerrero APS, Lee PC, Skokauskas N. 2018, 'Screening tools' chapter [7].

- *Family* is a child's first social group. It is a dynamic and complex system, in which members belong to and share the same social context. A child's first emotional exchanges and the construction of identity occur in the context of the family. Family structure and functioning is essential to help the child in adapting to life experiences, and ultimately aids the development of healthy attachment patterns. Parenting is the term used to describe the ways in which parents support the behavioural and mental health development of their children. Assessing the patient's family is especially relevant to child/adolescent mental health issues, as family problems (e.g., parenting style or parental marital conflict) can affect child development. In addition, sometimes child problematic behavior can elicit negative reactions of family members, which can start a cyclic conflictive relationship pattern. In these situations, evaluating the family system and the patterns of the family interactions is of paramount importance. In clinical work, several tools and frameworks have been used to perform family assessment, like the genogram [8], family life cycle assessment [9], and more structured tools like the Family APGAR [10]. These tools assess crucial characteristics of families such as interpersonal relationships, support, and affect. They can be very valuable in developing a comprehensive understanding of the child/adolescent's mental health issues in the context of the family, and in starting practical care.
- *Community* refers to a place where a child lives, goes to school, and plays. The environment (neighborhood, school, nature, local culture) plays an important role in mental health. Awareness of these factors is essential to developing solutions encompassing the entire system of care including other health or non-health public sectors (e.g., involving the educational system in cases of bullying, or discussing food/air/water safety with policymakers in cases of suspected intoxication/contamination syndromes). Community-level adversities (war, poverty, violence, climate changes, etc.) may be severe stressors and act as precipitating factors of mental disorders.

All in all, family doctors are usually able to generate an initial diagnostic hypothesis. The initial diagnostic hypothesis only needs to approximate the main psychiatric syndromes, i.e., the broad diagnostic category of the *Diagnostic and Statistical Manual* (DSM) of the American Psychiatric Association or International Classification of Diseases (ICD) in which the patient's mental health problems fit. It is noteworthy that International Classification of Primary Care (ICPC) proposes that mental health treatment may begin in primary care based on identifying broad diagnoses of problems rather than wait for nosology accuracy. Taking all this into account, and considering regional variations, as well as age specificities, the most common mental health conditions in children and adolescents are usually related to anxiety disorders, depressive disorders, ADHD, and disruptive behaviors [1]. These problems are frequently comorbid and have family and community roots, and should be the main target of general mental health care training of primary care providers.

Figure 10.1 tries to provide an overview of the process of assessing mental health problems in young people in primary care.

Initial problem management

The family doctor hypothesizes that Paulo is starting a first episode of major depression, and that this is related to the stressors he has experienced since the forced immigration process – a change of community, local difficulties in cultural and language adaptation, missing his father and grandparents, and the interruption of his plans to become an athlete. As well as referring the boy for psychotherapy, the family doctor wonders what else he could do, since it doesn't seem appropriate to start drug treatment at the moment. And he thinks that Paulo won't be the only child to come to him with these problems.

After the first syndromic hypothesis formulation, family doctors must consider additional tests or even a specialty care referral to obtain a definitive diagnosis. Established disorders must be treated according to standards of clinical management, which exceeds the scope of this chapter. However, there is much that the family doctor can do in the initial approach to treatment.

It is useful to remember the framework of PCM while considering general aspects of management. The *third component* of PCM states that a doctor must build a management plan in collaboration with the patient, negotiating what is possible. The *fourth component* of PCM requires that rapport be established during evaluation and management thus building trust and strengthening the doctor–patient relationship. Careful listening, an important element of this approach, must be especially empathetic at this point; that is, the doctor should employ a non-judgmental and compassionate stance to elicit the complaints of the patient and family and attempt to walk in their shoes, experience the feelings evoked by the situations shared, including potential reluctance to engage in proposed treatments.

In addition, there are many more structured interventions that can be delivered in mild cases, or even in more serious cases while awaiting specialized care. These so-called low intensity psychosocial interventions can be an important contribution of family doctors and primary care for youth mental health care. Individual interventions like behavioural activation [11], stress management [12] (including diaphragmatic breathing [13]) and

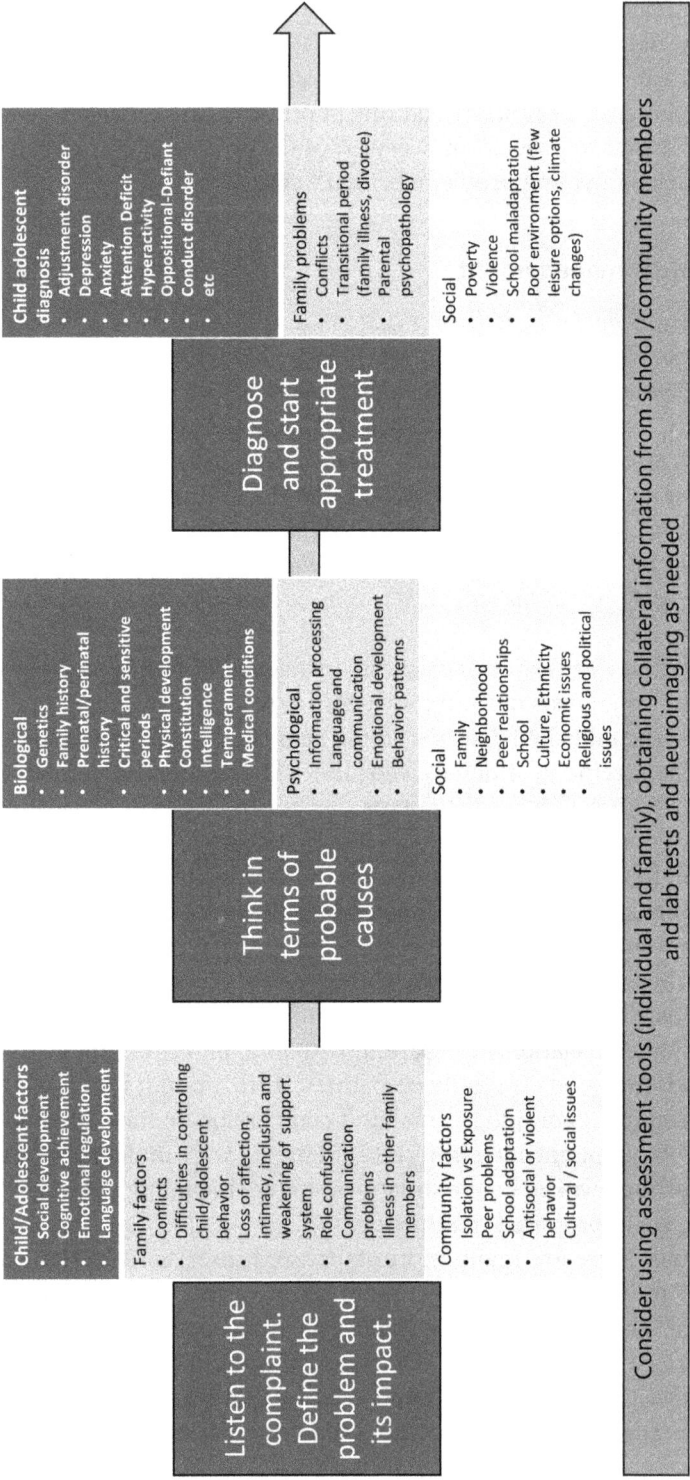

FIGURE 10.1 Schema of child/adolescent mental health problems comprehensive evaluation, built by the authors.

problem-solving skills [14] are examples of broadband transdiagnostic brief simple interventions that can be delivered effectively in primary care settings, even by non-doctors. Primary care providers also can be trained to perform family interventions like brief sessions to improve family communication, or parent training on fitting parenting style to child's temperament. Finally, community interventions could be the best choice in some cases; a growing approach in this regard is the Social Prescribing technique [15] – a tool that involves referring patients to non-clinical services, proposing involvement in a range of activities like volunteering, arts activities, gardening, befriending, cookery, and sports. Table 10.4 exemplifies selected low intensity interventions.

Community interventions have also been largely studied by The Blueprints for Healthy Youth Development Program (https://www.blueprintsprograms.org/), an American institution that provides a comprehensive registry of dozens of scientifically proven and scalable interventions that prevent or reduce the likelihood of antisocial behavior and promote a healthy course of youth development and adult maturity. This is a valuable resource to policymakers.

CURRENT ADDITIONAL THREATS TO MENTAL HEALTH – POST-PANDEMIC ERA/WAR/CLIMATE CHANGES

As mentioned, children's mental health has been related to multiple elements. Among them are environmental and sociocultural aspects that directly affect family dynamics and interpersonal interactions. Recently, post-pandemic slow economic recovery, current wars, and climate change have strongly affected families, resulting in severe problems for children, such as premature loss of loved ones, parental unemployment or forced migration.

During the COVID-19 pandemic all subjects experienced circumstances involving high levels of stress, anxiety, and feelings of helplessness and uncertainty. Early on it was suggested that, compared to adults, this pandemic would continue to have increased long-term adverse consequences on the mental health of children and adolescents [17]. In these age groups, the impact depends on different vulnerability factors including developmental age, educational level, special needs, previous mental health conditions, economic insecurity, among others. A meta-analysis of 29 studies with more than 80,000 participants has estimated that during the first year of the pandemic one in four young people worldwide experienced clinically elevated depressive symptoms, while one in five young people experienced clinically elevated anxiety symptoms. These combined estimates are twice as high as pre-pandemic estimates. Prevalence rates were higher later in the pandemic, in older adolescents and in girls. Based on these results, a greater need for

TABLE 10.4 Some brief interventions for youth mental health care in primary care

Interventions	Problem	Technique	Example
Individual	Excessive worries and anxiety agitation	Diaphragmatic breathing	Teach deep breathing – slowly inhaling for 3 seconds, holding for 3 seconds, exhaling for 3 seconds, not moving the thorax, only the belly. Practice it for 3 minutes, 3 times each day, and more sessions as needed. Practice and discuss its effects with the patient. Show videos to help [13].
Familial	Disruptive, aggressive behavior	Parent training	Teach parents about the temperament dimensions proposed by Thomas and Chess [16] (innate, non-voluntary individual characteristics like level of activity, adjustment profile, reactivity, biological rhythm regularity, approach/ withdrawal pattern, persistence, intensity, mood, distractibility, responsiveness threshold). Talk about the need to keep in mind that confrontation can worsen the problem, and help parents to find alternative ways to teach youth how to cope with stress.
Community	Low mood / depression	Social prescribing	Keep available a list of non-clinical services in the neighborhood. Make shared decisions with the child/adolescent about what activity to start and follow the adhesion and impact in mental health. Start low, go slow but forward.

All the techniques above must be revised periodically, to correct application and adherence.

Source: Compiled by the authors.

mental health care is expected, highlighting the importance of resource allocation to address child and adolescent mental health problems [18].

Further, armed conflict generates significant repercussions in the general population, and various psychopathological manifestations in children and adolescents. In 2018, the United Nations Children's Fund (UNICEF) noted that episodes of extreme violence against children and adolescents are common in armed conflicts, either by using them as human shields or by recruiting, abducting or sexually abusing them [19]. The acute and chronic effects of armed conflict on children's health and well-being are among the greatest violations of children's rights in the 21st century. The intensity, suddenness, and duration of armed conflicts are associated with the appearance of psychopathology – especially of the affective type – and impairment of important different functional skills and capacities in the child or adolescent. It is suggested that vulnerability increases the earlier that children are exposed to armed conflicts, and it is worsened with deaths in or forced separation from their families. A review of the literature [20] showed that out of 72 publications of studies conducted between 1989 and 2018, the negative consequences on mental health in the pre-conflict, conflict, and post-conflict period are in the spectrum of depression, anxiety, and post-traumatic stress. Youth also presented with attention difficulties, experiences of insecurity, aggressiveness, cognitive distortions, and use of psychoactive substances. This review pointed out that in the period prior to the war, mainly anticipatory somatic symptoms were observed (e.g., headaches and other physical pain) as well as manifestations such as fear and hopelessness linked to the possibility of migration or family disintegration. During the period in which the war conflict develops, different manifestations occur, the most frequent being enuresis, fear, sadness, aggressiveness, hyperactivity, and inattention. Aggressiveness may remain beyond the end of the war conflict. Difficulties in the relationship with parents and decreased social skills were also observed. It also noted the presence of adjustment disorders, depression, anxiety and, to a greater extent, post-traumatic stress disorder with secondary fears of family separation, exaggerated reaction to noise, nervous states, aggression and agitation, excessive crying, sleep problems or anxious activation. The same review found that symptoms differ according to the duration, exposure to or escalation of the conflict. In the post-conflict period, the resolution of symptomatology is linked to resilience and the presence of protective factors such as family support and accompaniment, and the social support provided by peers, school, and community. Furthermore, in these circumstances, the mental health conditions of adult caregivers was a very important factor since it influenced the development of psychopathology in children.

Finally, climate change is widely acknowledged as a current global public health crisis. The 20th century saw rapid industrialization driven by fossil fuel use in the global north. This development resulted in increasing atmospheric CO_2 levels (from 285 parts per million [ppm] in the pre-industrial area to 407 in 2018), with consequent sharp increases in global temperatures. These climate-related events have had far-reaching impacts. Climate change characterized by uncertain intensity, duration, and frequency of weather patterns contributes to impaired physical and mental health as well as psychosocial and economic insecurity. For instance, prolonged drought can increase environmental dust, alter disease patterns, pollen, and water-borne diseases, and food and water insecurity. Thus, climate change influences pediatric mental health through the direct neuropsychiatric consequences of increased heat, aeroallergens, greenhouse gases, and other pollutants as well as indirect consequences of trauma related to severe weather events (e.g., drought, famine, floods, heatwaves, wildfires) and resultant disruptions (e.g., geopolitical conflict, forced migration, human trafficking). The pediatric mental health consequences range from increased risk of anxiety, depression, post-traumatic stress disorder to substance use disorders and suicidal ideation. Notably, climate change disproportionately affects vulnerable populations such as youth and those with pre-existing mental illness. Children's immature physiology and dependence on adult caregivers [21] make them uniquely susceptible to the health effects of climate change. In fact, the 2021 US Surgeon General's report acknowledges climate change as one of the driving factors in the current pediatric mental health crisis [22]. Youth also experience significant non-pathological emotions (anxiety, fear, anger, guilt, and grief) related to the climate crisis more so than adults, which may be collectively characterized as 'climate distress' (also called eco-anxiety). Additionally, as healthcare providers, it is important to consider climate change in the context of (1) the risk of mental health care delivery disruption and (2) the potential for emissions mitigation as the healthcare sector accounts for 8.5% of total US greenhouse gas emissions. From a health equity perspective, climate change is a threat amplifier that disproportionately targets populations already impacted by racial, socio-economic, and political discrimination. For instance, vulnerable populations in the global south, especially children, bear the brunt of higher levels of toxic exposure and lower levels of resilience to climate change. This is even though much of climate change has been precipitated by the actions of the global north in their indiscriminate exploitation of natural resources.

All this considered, primary care physicians should provide timely care for potential mental health issues in climate disasters. Migration/

displacement-specific mental issues, trauma-related disorders, and grief support deserve a special highlight.

Initiatives to mitigate immigration/displacement, poverty, trauma, and distress

As the world witnesses natural and manmade disasters, families and entire populations have been displaced. This forced migration is innately traumatic. The attendant issues of diminished access to education, healthcare, safe housing for children and employment opportunities for parents have a powerful impact on migrant and refugee families. Additionally, discrimination and anti-immigrant policies magnify immigrant health disparities. There is evidence that xenophobia, bullying of immigrant youth and discriminatory harassment by peers at school result in internalizing symptoms, such as depression [23].

By 2015, an estimated 244 million people lived in a country other than their country of birth [24]. By 2021 almost 89.3 million people were forcibly displaced according to the United Nations [25]. Complex migratory journeys, fragmented social networks, experiences of racism or discrimination, social unrest, and interruptions in children's social and educational development, pre- or post-migration traumatic experiences linked to war, persecution or violence increase mental health risks [26–28]. Although the 'healthy immigrant effect' touts immigrants having better health than the population of the host country, their health invariably worsens over time. Refugees usually arrive in worse general state of health compared to immigrants [29]. The impact of war on children has several implications: immediate responses to stress, increased risk of specific mental disorders, distress due to forced separation from parents, and fear for personal and family safety [30]. Young immigrants are at greater risk of suffering from psychopathological disorders like post-traumatic stress disorder, depression, conduct disorder, and problems linked to substance abuse. During migration, many young people are separated from their parents and lose the emotional, physical, and financial support of their family. Unaccompanied minors and children with unstable living situations are at increased risk of mental health problems. Unaccompanied children or unaccompanied refugee minors refer to forcibly displaced children and youth under the age of 18 separated from both parents and not in the care of an adult. They are a vulnerable subgroup with high levels of anguish and depression [30].

Although, on the other hand, many young immigrants do well upon arrival and some surpass their peers in their country of origin in academic aspirations and achievements, in the post-migration phase young people often face significant and multiple stressors, as shown in Table 10.5.

TABLE 10.5 Immigration-related stressors posing mental health risks

Cultural	• Linguistic and cultural barriers
Health services	• Systemic access barriers • Disease behavior • Stigma about mental health care and fear of negative repercussions from said care • Children and adolescents are often referred and taken to treatment by caregivers and may not understand or agree with the decision to seek therapy services
Family	• Effect of family structure, acculturation, and intergenerational conflict • Immigrant families from different cultural backgrounds may know less about how therapy works and what the roles of the parent, partner, child, adolescent, and mental health professional
Social	• Facilitation or impediment of adaptation • Social integration by the receiving society. Post-migration factors, including the quality of reception and support in the country of asylum, are important predictors of long-term outcomes • Living in underserved areas with poor access to mental health services, once this correlates to higher rates of suicide, depression, and substance use • Poverty, which is associated with a wide range of detrimental health impacts, negative educational outcomes, and adverse long-term social and psychological outcomes • Violence against immigrant children includes anti-immigration measures or detention, forced child labor, bullying, domestic violence, xenophobia, and child trafficking

Many strategies to improve the delivery of mental health services can be implemented as family or parent interventions. Furthermore, many of these strategies propose early intervention to improve the quality of life of children as well as treatment and continuous monitoring for those who require it [28]. Psychosocial and mental health interventions for immigrant children should be multi-level, specifically targeted to the needs of the child, trauma-informed, and focused on extant strengths and resilience building [30]. Table 10.6 shows elements on which interventions can be carried out to improve immigrant/displaced child mental health.

Identifying and managing youth with specific trauma-related disorders

According to the DSM-5 [45], traumatic events are 'events that involve actual or threatened death or serious injury, or a threat to the physical integrity of oneself or others'. Besides direct exposure to a traumatic event,

TABLE 10.6 Interventions to ameliorate immigration/forced displacement effects on mental health

Element	Impact	Intervention	Actions
Resilience building	Exerts a protective effect against stressful events, preventing the development of psychological disorders.	Promote four competencies: Social competence, problem solving, autonomy, and positive experiences for the future [31].	Systematic screening with holistic management that includes clinical approaches and the supplementation of basic needs [32].
		Perform interventions in working memory.	By addressing preparation, execution, regulation, and adjustments of behavior, emotion, and cognition, it provides temporary storage and allows the manipulation of information necessary for language comprehension, learning, and reasoning that is vital in child development [33].
Social support	Networks outside the family can play an important role for the mental health of Unaccompanied Refugee Minors (URM) who face great challenges [32, 34–36].	Social, economic, and cultural integration in host societies [24].	Social support provided by people from the same cultural background, the nuclear family, extended family members, peers (greater peer support in adolescence predicts lower levels of depression and promotes mental health), and professionals (e.g., social workers, teachers, mentors, coaches) [34].
		Community-based models: Flexible, address complex needs, and situated within communities [24].	Work with community organizations: immigrant youth who live in communities with a high proportion of immigrants of the same origin adapt better, in part because they have positive role models, a greater sense of ethnic pride, and social support, which can be protective against stressors of poverty, discrimination, and racism. Likewise, faith communities provide support in adaptation. It is recommended to have a list of community resources for specific needs (e.g., housing, food, language courses, social support) and the ethnocultural groups that these resources represent [27]. School interventions for children and adolescents to reach rural populations. They may include group and/or individual services for children and adolescents [37].
Cultural	Strengthening cultural competence.	Intercultural understanding [27].	Cultural competence in the receiving culture and heritage. Both are important for children to develop a sense of belonging [38, 39].

(Continued)

TABLE 10.6 Interventions to ameliorate immigration/forced displacement effects on mental health (*Continued*)

Element	Impact	Intervention	Actions
Regarding mental health	Holistic productive and preventive approach to services that are flexible, affordable, accessible, and culturally and linguistically appropriate.	Doctor–patient communication [27]. Use of interpreters (in person, when possible) and cultural agents.	Build rapport and establish the truth, expressing empathy [38]. To avoid a family member (especially a child) from taking on the role which causes loss of confidentiality and a greater burden for children (parentification) [24, 27, 38]. Prior and subsequent meetings with the interpreter should be held to improve patient care. During the interview: introduce yourself and the interpreter; explain the function it will have; discuss with the patient about confidentiality; obtain patient consent; avoid jargon, use clear words with colloquial language; speak slowly, so that the translation can take place; clarify responses related to non-verbal language; and provide space for the patient's questions and concerns [24, 27, 38].
		Actions and policies, by facilitating sleep, self-confidence, and concentration [26].	Addressing depressive symptoms and anxiety [26]. The personalization of services. Implementing the '3ps Approach' (preventive, predictive, and personalized medicine). The first refers to the exploration of the factors that predispose the sleep disorder, prevention focuses on education about sleep hygiene and knowledge about the consequences of insomnia. Personalization refers to aspects that have already been discussed (consider language, easy access to the service, early treatment) [40]. Image rehearsal therapies can be used for nightmares and nightmare disorders related to post-traumatic stress disorder, cognitive-behavioural therapy, to name a few [41, 42].
		In rural areas	The therapist can begin using telehealth, scheduled telephone contact or email correspondence. Especially to evaluate and diagnose children [37].

Family	Family cohesion and the perception of parental support are negatively associated with mental health problems in children and adolescents, and act as protective factors against stress. Family cohesion becomes a predictor of the mental health of refugee children [34].	Creation of programs for parents.	The family develops social networks, as well as learning about well-being and raising children [24]. Psychoeducate families in the scope of mental health care [30, 37].
Individual		Perform play therapy.	For the expression of conflicts and anxiety in the context of a therapeutic relationship, such as artistic techniques, playing with dolls, puppet playing, storytelling, board games, etc. [43].
		Crisis intervention. It is a quick and brief collaboration to promote resilience and help the person in their survival and resolve the crisis in the face of any event or condition, individual or community. Crisis intervention with children involves considering the family's systemic vision, the family context, its history, and its family constitution [44].	Promote social support: Where they get affection, comfort, affirmation, advice, and assistance. Drive away isolation and alienation. All for the benefit of resolving the crisis [44]. Connect children with other children to promote a sense of community in the face of a disaster. The children are placed in pairs. It can begin with a phrase: 'from my heart to yours, I hope you are well', while pointing to your heart (foot to foot, hand to hand, shoulder to shoulder, etc.) and that of your partner [44].

(Continued)

TABLE 10.6 Interventions to ameliorate immigration/forced displacement effects on mental health *(Continued)*

Element	Impact	Intervention	Actions
Individual (continued)			Give meaning: With various activities (drawing, speaking, playing, sculpting, singing, writing), they tell their story that allows us to see the crisis from a cognitive perspective, give shape to the harshness of that reality and find possible solutions. This gives the person identity and becomes part of their family legacy. It allows you to reaffirm your beliefs, guide decisions and offer comfort. They move from the narrative of a crisis to the story of a survivor [44].
			Survivor's Diary: It is related to satisfaction in the process of transforming your life into words. Narrative therapy helps the child rewrite their story, not only in terms of the crisis, but also their stories of survival. You can know the history, the impact, and the way they go through this challenge [30, 44].

Source: Compiled by the authors.

the DSM-5 also includes witnessing a traumatic event, or learning that the traumatic event(s) occurred to a close family member or close friend, and/or extreme and repeated exposure to aversive details of the traumatic events. Post-trauma, children may show signs of regression i.e., loss of previously acquired skills. Exposure to acute trauma (abuse, sudden loss of family member, domestic violence, war, natural disaster) can result in a host of childhood mental health issues ranging from short-lasting acute stress disorders (lasting two days to one month) to the more severe and longer lasting post-traumatic stress disorders (lasting more than a month), depression, panic disorder, specific phobias related to the trauma, as well as behavioural and attentional problems. In terms of interventions, debriefing is no longer routinely recommended for children and adolescents exposed to trauma. The consensus is to provide psychological first aid, a structured technique consisting of education about normal reactions to trauma, and delivering basic medical and safety needs, for example, shelter, food, social support, and referral as needed. For post-traumatic stress disorder, time-limited therapies like trauma-focused cognitive-behavioural therapy (TF-CBT) based on the principles of exposure and remodeling of cognitive processes have proved efficacy in children [46]. When culturally adapted, TF-CBT is effective in treating trauma-related symptoms and improving psychosocial functioning in children and adolescents in low- and middle-income countries [47]. A system of care approach that utilizes a trauma-informed lens is paramount to address adverse childhood experiences and trauma. The family being the first system of care for youth, family interventions that are trauma informed (i.e., reinforce a sense of safety, trust, collaboration, and empowerment) are key in the treatment of trauma.

Helping children and adolescents deal with grief

Grief is a normal and expected reaction to a loss of any kind (traditionally death but can be others) and the process that the person goes through to adapt to a new life situation after such loss [48]. The magnitude of the pain experienced when facing the loss will depend on the meaning it has for the subject. Kübler-Ross [49] described the best-known model for the elaboration of grief, which consists of five stages: denial, anger, bargaining, depression, and acceptance. These stages may or may not be consecutive and in children especially it can be oscillating.

With the loss of a significant emotional figure for a child or adolescent (either by death or abandonment), the severity of the symptoms usually requires significant support from their environment, and may even require professional support, especially considering that adult caregivers may also be grieving (double grieving). In children and adolescents, the manifestations may be delayed in time. Therefore, it is important to check whether the bereavement is evolving adequately and to avoid possible complications [50]. Symptoms are usually comparable to those of a major depressive episode (sadness, anger, longing, guilt, etc.), with significant compromise, discomfort, and functional impairment. What gives it the characteristic of 'normal' and not pathological is that in this case the symptoms arise in response to the loss of an important loved one (parents, siblings, grandparents, etc.). It is postulated that internal factors such as resilience and external factors such as family and social support are variables that allow the processing of the loss in an adequate manner [51]. How adults convey their own perceptions of death and their own bereavement experiences to children is important for children's bereavement experiences [52].

In the DSM-5, bereavement is not listed as a mental disorder but is placed in the category of additional disorders that may require clinical attention. A grieving child or adolescent may become depressed if they do not have sufficient family or professional support or may present the characteristics of a post-traumatic stress disorder when the death occurs in a violent manner. For this reason, it is important to listen to them and help them process the loss. The intensity and prolongation of the manifestations can mean that normal grief has turned into complicated grief although there is no unanimous agreement. For example, if grief is prolonged for more than six months or if psychotic symptoms or other serious signs appear, it is an indicator that it is no longer a normal grief process and requires specialized care. If the child or adolescent or the family requests specialist care, referral is also important.

SERVICE DELIVERY – IMPLICATIONS FOR PRIMARY CARE PRACTICE

Child and adolescent psychiatry, a specialized field of medicine, is an independent specialty in some countries. This means that physicians need a very broad knowledge to help patients without doing harm (e.g., prescribing inappropriate drugs, or not detecting serious conditions). On the other hand, it is well known that the world has a dearth of specialized professionals, including child/adolescent psychologists and multidisciplinary teams that are scarce even in developed countries. Family doctors and primary care teams are especially well positioned for early detection and intervention in youth mental disorders. However, innovative workforce strategies and capacity building are essential. With momentum for these efforts increasing on a global scale, the time is right for joint efforts to further develop these approaches in systems of care.

Integrated care experiences

Collaboration between family physicians and pediatricians is a crucial aspect of primary care in many settings. This partnership ensures comprehensive and coordinated care, particularly for children and families. By working together, family physicians and pediatricians can address a wide range of health needs, leverage their unique expertise, and promote continuity of care across the lifespan. This important topic deserves careful consideration to enhance the quality and effectiveness of primary healthcare delivery. It is important to keep in mind that the integration between family doctors and mental health specialists must always include the pediatrician, either as the first specialist to whom the family doctor refers or as part of a team in complex cases. In addition to specialized knowledge in childhood, which may already be sufficient in most cases, the pediatrician will also benefit from working with mental health specialists, developing their skills to deal with problems in this area.

Several integrated care models between primary care providers (family doctors or pediatricians) and mental health services have been tested around the world, and include specific programs for youth care [53]. Child Psychiatry Access Programs (that provide consultation to pediatric primary care providers) in the United States are an example of a model of coordinated care that maximizes the mental health workforce by empowering pediatric primary care providers to treat mild to moderate mental illness. This system of care approach has been proposed as a solution to improve access to care in underserved areas that are especially plagued by the workforce shortage [54].

Tele-mental health opportunities

Another successful modality to improve access to care in underserved areas has been the use of telemedicine (by phone as well as by audiovisual platforms) at various levels of care i.e., inpatient, outpatient, emergency room and even in Child Psychiatry Access Programs [55]. This has proven to be a scalable solution with proven provider and patient satisfaction in developing nations like India [56]. Tele-mental health care may allow for a deeper understanding when seeing children in their home settings, often offering the possibility of meeting other family members thereby making connections that would not otherwise be possible. This technology may thus present opportunities to weave in family work and the possibility of gathering collateral information and educating school staff during the 'medication visit'. With the increasing availability and convenience of video conferencing technology, promotion of tele-mental health through funding, advocacy, and training would allow for widespread use of this service delivery model. For instance, Saudi Arabia is piloting the use of smartphone applications and a network to connect specialized facilities with primary care centers and hospitals in underserved areas. In low-resource areas, assistance with technology and Wi-Fi access would reduce some of the barriers to tele-mental health.

Teleconferences among professionals have proven efficacy as a teaching model and in improving the quality of care. One of the most successful initiatives worldwide is the Extension for Community Healthcare Outcomes (ECHO) Project of the University of New Mexico in the United States (https://projectecho.unm.edu/). The ECHO Project is a model of tele-mentoring based on 90–120-minute case discussions that help distant sites to understand and treat complex clinical problems. ECHO sessions are structured as follows: participants present real (anonymized) cases to the specialists and to each other for discussion and recommendations. There are currently programs in more than 50 countries, several dedicated to child/adolescent mental health, like the Ontario Mental Health CAMH and University of Toronto, in Canada, and the Autism hub of the University of Missouri.

Education and advocacy to address workforce shortages and access to care

Specific educational/training programs have been proposed by important international organizations to foster workforce development in youth mental health care. The International Association of Child and Adolescent Psychiatry and Allied Professionals (IACAPAP) has developed and displayed in its website valuable resources like a free e-textbook translated into several languages, as well as practical strategies to face current crises like pandemics and war. Additionally, IACAPAP has offered a Massive Open Online Course (MOOC) 'designed to meet the basic educational needs of people interested in child and adolescent mental health such as nurses, community health workers, teachers, general practitioners, medical students, adult psychiatrists, and parents'. The course is simple, user friendly and each session includes a 20-minute video (see Further Reading and e-Resources). The World Psychiatric Association also has developed several educational initiatives like COVID-19 and Ukraine War freely available in its website (www.wpanet.org), as well as an educational portal with multimedia content about mental health problems in children for non-specialist providers. Finally, the World Health Organization has also been working in this field, especially developing materials for non-mental health specialized professionals, like the well-known mhGAP Program, which recently developed a specific module for child and adolescent care.

Finally, integration of mental health into the primary care residency program curriculum has been debated worldwide. Recently the status of mental health training curricula in family medicine residency was surveyed internationally, and 'the results revealed that many academic societies have created competency lists and curriculum guidelines for mental health training; however, the implementation varied' [57]. Based on the arguments presented so far, special emphasis on child/adolescent mental health care is needed in future discussions.

RECOMMENDATIONS

- Keep in mind local child/adolescent mental health care epidemiology and professional gap.
- Include in permanent medical education practical principles of approaching the most common mental health problems by age, with an emphasis on assessment and initial management.
- Discuss with healthcare teams recent findings about new threats to youth mental health coming from current global problems – post-pandemic era issues, regional wars, and climate change.
- Present options to improve access to care through systems rethinking, especially through telemedicine use, collaborative care models with pediatrics and psychiatry, and education/training of primary care workers in this field.

FURTHER READING AND e-RESOURCES

- IACAPAP (see e-textbook and MOOC)
  - https://iacapap.org/
- World Psychiatric Association (WPA) (see Educational Portal)
  - https://www.wpanet.org/
- American Academy of Child and Adolescent Psychiatry (AACAP) (see Practice Parameters)
  - https://www.aacap.org/
- Children & War Foundation
  - https://www.childrenandwar.org/
- mhGap 2.0
  - https://www.who.int/teams/mental-health-and-substance-use/treatment-care/mental-health-gap-action-programme/evidence-centre

REFERENCES

1. Polanczyk GV, Salum GA, Sugaya LS, et al. Annual research review: a meta-analysis of the worldwide prevalence of mental disorders in children and adolescents. J Child Psychol Psychiatry. 2015;56:345–365. https://doi.org/10.1111/jcpp.12381
2. Kessler RC, Berglund P, Demler O, et al. Lifetime prevalence and age-of-onset distributions of DSM-IV disorders in the national comorbidity survey replication. Arch Gen Psychiatry. 2005;62:593–602. https://doi.org/10.1001/archpsyc.62.6.593

3. Shaligram D, Bernstein B, DeJong SM, et al. "Building" the twenty-first century child and adolescent psychiatrist. Acad Psychiatry. 2022;46:75–81. https://doi.org/10.1007/s40596-022-01594-4

4. Kramer T, Garralda ME. Child and adolescent mental health problems in primary care. Adv Psychiatr Treat. 2000;6. https://doi.org/10.1192/apt.6.4.287

5. Stewart M, Brown JB, Weston WW, et al. Patient-Centered Medicine: Transforming the Clinical Method. 3rd ed. 2013. CRC Press, London. https://doi.org/10.1201/b20740

6. Shaffer DR, Kipp K. Developmental Psychology: Childhood and Adolescence. 7th ed. Australia: Wadsworth/Thomson 2007.

7. Anthony AP, Lee PC, Skokauskas N. Pediatric Consultation-liaison Psychiatry a Global, Healthcare Systems-Focused, and Problem-Based Approach. 2018. Springer, Cham, Switzerland. https://doi.org/10.1007/978-3-319-89488-1

8. Waters I, Watson W, Wetzel W. Genograms. Practical tools for family physicians. Can Fam Physician. 1994;40:282–287.

9. Roberts L. The Family Life Cycle in Medical Practice. In The Family in Medical Practice. 1987. Springer, New York, NY. https://doi.org/10.1007/978-1-4612-4642-8_4

10. Smilkstein G. The family APGAR: a proposal for a family function test and its use by physicians. J Fam Pract. 1978 Jun;6(6):1231–1239. PMID: 660126.

11. Martin F, Oliver T. Behavioral activation for children and adolescents: a systematic review of progress and promise. Eur Child Adolesc Psychiatry. 2019;28:427–441. https://doi.org/10.1007/s00787-018-1126-z

12. Zisopoulou T, Varvogli L. Stress management methods in children and adolescents: past, present, and future. Horm Res Paediatr. 2023;96:97–107. https://doi.org/10.1159/000526946

13. The Mindfulness Teacher. Belly Breathing: Mindfulness for Children. 2020. Video available in https://www.youtube.com/watch?v=RiMb2Bw4Ae8

14. Stewart RA. Review of problem solving in child and adolescent psychotherapy: a skills-based, collaborative approach. Sch Soc Work J. 2014;38.

15. Bertotti M, Hayes D, Berry V, et al. Social prescribing for children and young people. Lancet Child Adolesc Health. 2022;6:835–837. https://doi.org/10.1016/S2352-4642(22)00248-6

16. Chess S, Thomas A. Temperament: Theory and Practice. Psychology Press 1996. Brunner/Mazel, New York.

17. Shen K, Yang Y, Wang T, et al. Diagnosis, treatment, and prevention of 2019 novel coronavirus infection in children: experts' consensus statement. World J Pediatr. 2020;16:223–231. https://doi.org/10.1007/s12519-020-00343-7

18. Racine N, McArthur BA, Cooke JE, et al. Global prevalence of depressive and anxiety symptoms in children and adolescents during COVID-19: a meta-analysis. JAMA Pediatr. 2021;175:1142–1150. https://doi.org/10.1001/jamapediatrics.2021.2482

19. England J. World has failed to protect children in conflict in 2018: UNICEF. 2018 December 27. Available on https://www.unicef.org/eca/press-releases/world-has-failed-protect-children-conflict-2018.

20. Piñeros-Ortiz S, Moreno-Chaparro J, Garzón-Orjuela N, et al. Mental health consequences of armed conflicts in children and adolescents: an overview of literature reviews. Biomedica. 2021 Sep 22;41(3):424–448. English, Spanish. doi: 10.7705/biomedica.5447. PMID: 34559491; PMCID: PMC8525875.

21. Perera F, Nadeau K. Climate change, fossil-fuel pollution, and children's health. N Engl J Med. 2022 Jun 16;386(24):2303–2314. https://doi.org/10.1056/NEJMra2117706. PMID: 35704482.

22. Office of the Surgeon General (OSG). Protecting Youth Mental Health: The U.S. Surgeon General's Advisory [Internet]. Washington (DC): US Department of Health and Human Services; 2021.

23. Marks AK, McKenna JL, Coll CG. National immigration receiving contexts: a critical aspect of native-born, immigrant, and refugee youth well-being. Eur Psychol. 2018;23. https://doi.org/10.1027/1016-9040/a000311

24. Salami B, Salma J, Hegadoren K. Access and utilization of mental health services for immigrants and refugees: perspectives of immigrant service providers. Int J Ment Health Nurs. 2019;28:152–161. https://doi.org/10.1111/inm.12512

25. United Nations High Commissioner for Refugees. Global Trends Forced Displacement in 2021. UNHCR Global Trends. 2021. 48. https://doi.org/10.18356/9789211065992

26. Buchcik J, Kovach V, Adedeji A. Mental health outcomes and quality of life of Ukrainian refugees in Germany. Health Qual Life Outcomes. 2023;21. https://doi.org/10.1186/s12955-023-02101-5

27. Kirmayer LJ, Narasiah L, Munoz M, Rashid M, Ryder AG, Guzder J, Hassan G, Rousseau C, Pottie K; Canadian Collaboration for Immigrant and Refugee Health (CCIRH). Common mental health problems in immigrants and refugees: general approach in primary care. CMAJ. 2011 Sep 6;183(12):E959–E967. https://doi.org/10.1503/cmaj.090292

28. Berkowitz SJ, Marans S. Crisis Intervention: Secondary Prevention for Children Exposed to Violence. In Children Exposed to Violence. In M. M. Feerick & G. B. Silverman (Eds.), Children exposed to violence. 2006;137–158. Paul H. Brookes Publishing Co., Towson, Maryland.

29. Woodgate RL, Busolo DS, Crockett M, et al. A qualitative study on African immigrant and refugee families' experiences of accessing primary health care services in Manitoba, Canada: It's not easy! Int J Equity Health. 2017;16:5. https://doi.org/10.1186/s12939-016-0510-x

30. Mohwinkel LM, Nowak AC, Kasper A, et al. Gender differences in the mental health of unaccompanied refugee minors in Europe: a systematic review. BMJ Open. 2018;8:e022389. https://doi.org/10.1136/bmjopen-2018-022389

31. Solà-Sales S, Pérez-González N, Van Hoey J, Iborra-Marmolejo I, Beneyto-Arrojo MJ, Moret-Tatay C. The role of resilience for migrants and refugees' mental health in times of COVID-19. Healthcare (Basel). 2021 Aug 30;9(9):1131. https://doi.org/10.3390/healthcare9091131

32. Bapolisi AM, Song SJ, Kesande C, et al. Post-traumatic stress disorder, psychiatric comorbidities and associated factors among refugees in Nakivale camp in southwestern Uganda. BMC Psychiatry. 2020;20:53. https://doi.org/10.1186/s12888-020-2480-1

33. Ramírez L, Lizarazo Y, Bonilla-Cruz N, et al. Estrategias de intervención en la memoria de trabajo en niños y niñas sobrevivientes del desplazamiento forzado y la crisis fronteriza en Venezuela. Arch Venez Farmacol Ter. 2020;39:98–104.

34. Sierau S, Schneider E, Nesterko Y, et al. Alone, but protected? Effects of social support on mental health of unaccompanied refugee minors. Eur Child Adolesc Psychiatry. 2019;28:769–780. https://doi.org/10.1007/s00787-018-1246-5

35. Giannopoulou I, Mourloukou L, Efstathiou V, et al. Mental health of unaccompanied refugee minors in Greece living 'in limbo'. Psychiatriki. 2022;33:219–227. https://doi.org/10.22365/jpsych.2022.074

36. von Werthern M, Grigorakis G, Vizard E. The mental health and wellbeing of unaccompanied refugee minors (URMs). Child Abuse Negl. 2019;98:104146. https://doi.org/10.1016/j.chiabu.2019.104146

37. Smalley KB, Yancey CT, Warren JC, et al. Rural mental health and psychological treatment: a review for practitioners. J Clin Psychol. 2010;66. https://doi.org/10.1002/jclp.20688

38. Kroening ALH, Dawson-Hahn E. Health considerations for immigrant and refugee children. Adv Pediatr. 2019;66. https://doi.org/10.1016/j.yapd.2019.04.003

39. Oppedal B, Keles S, Cheah C, et al. Culture competence and mental health across different immigrant and refugee groups. BMC Public Health. 2020;20:292. https://doi.org/10.1186/s12889-020-8398-1

40. Richter K, Baumgärtner L, Niklewski G, et al. Sleep disorders in migrants and refugees: a systematic review with implications for personalized medical approach. EPMA J. 2020;11:251–260. https://doi.org/10.1007/s13167-020-00205-2

41. Gill P, Fraser E, Tran TTD, et al. Psychosocial treatments for nightmares in adults and children: a systematic review. BMC Psychiatry. 2023;23:283. https://doi.org/10.1186/s12888-023-04703-1

42. Sandahl H, Jennum P, Baandrup L, et al. Treatment of sleep disturbances in trauma-affected refugees: study protocol for a randomised controlled trial. Trials. 2017;18:520. https://doi.org/10.1186/s13063-017-2260-5

43. Webb, N. B. Play Therapy Crisis Intervention with Children. In N. B. Webb (Ed.), Play Therapy with Children in Crisis: Individual, Group, and Family Treatment (2nd ed., pp. 39–46). Guilford Press, New York, 1999.

44. Echterling LG, Stewart AL. Creative crisis Intervention Techniques with Children and Families. In Creative Interventions with Traumatized Children, 2nd ed. 2015. The Guilford Press, New York.

45. Association AP. Diagnostic and statistical manual of mental disorders: DSM-5-TR. 2022.

46. De Arellano MAR, Lyman R, Jobe-Shields L, et al. Trauma-focused cognitive-behavioral therapy for children and adolescents: assessing the evidence. Psych Servs. 2014;65. https://doi.org/10.1176/appi.ps.201300255

47. Thomas FC, Puente-Duran S, Mutschler C, et al. Trauma-focused cognitive behavioral therapy for children and youth in low-and middle-income countries: a systematic review. Child Adolesc Ment Health. 2022;27:146–160. https://doi.org/10.1111/camh.12435

48. García A, Rodríguez M, Brito P, et al. Duelo adaptativo, no adaptativo y continuidad de vínculos. Ene. 2021;15:1–26.

49. Kübler-Ross E. On death and dying. New York: Macmillan Company 1969.

50. Barreto P, De la Torre O, Pérez-Marín M. Detección de duelo complicado. Psicooncologia (Pozuelo de Alarcon). 2013;9. https://doi.org/10.5209/rev_PSIC.2013.v9.n2-3.40902

51. Mallon, B. Working with Bereaved Children and Young People. SAGE Publications Ltd 2011. SAGE Publications, London. https://doi.org/10.4135/9781446251881

52. de Andrade ML. Depois do temporal: um estudo psicodinâmico sobre a criança enlutada e seus pais. 2013. https://doi.org/10.11606/D.59.2013.tde-12022014-084235

53. Shaligram D, Skokauskas N, Aragones E, et al. International perspective on integrated care models in child and adult mental health. Int Rev Psychiatry. 2022;34:101–117. https://doi.org/10.1080/09540261.2022.2059346

54. Sullivan K, George P, Horowitz K. Addressing national workforce shortages by funding child psychiatry access programs. Pediatrics. 2021;147:e20194012. https://doi.org/10.1542/PEDS.2019-4012

55. Hilt RJ. Telemedicine for child collaborative or integrated care. Child Adolesc Psychiatr Clin N Am. 2017;26:637–645. https://doi.org/10.1016/j.chc.2017.05.001

56. Kommu JVS, Sharma E, Ramtekkar U. Telepsychiatry for mental health service delivery to children and adolescents. Indian J Psychol Med. 2020;42:46S–52S. https://doi.org/10.1177/0253717620959256

57. Kawada S, Moriya J, Wakabayashi H, et al. Mental health training in family medicine residencies: international curriculum overview. J Gen Fam Med. 2023;24:63–71. https://doi.org/10.1002/jgf2.608

Index

For Product Safety Concerns and Information please contact our EU
representative GPSR@taylorandfrancis.com
Taylor & Francis Verlag GmbH, Kaufingerstraße 24, 80331 München, Germany

9 781032 754260